The Medicinal Power of Food

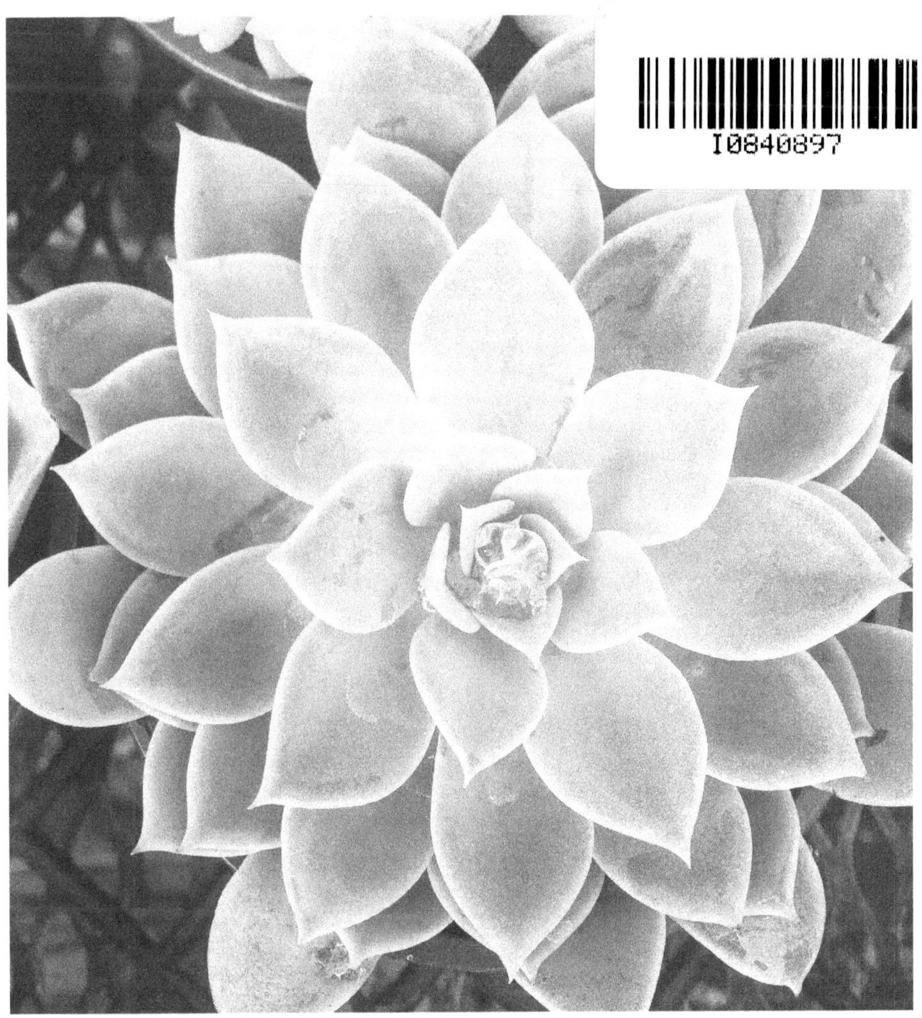

A beginners guide to healing with food / simple plant based recipes

Kyra Ann Hermann
Certified Family Herbalist

THE MEDICINAL POWER OF FOOD

Author & Photographer:
Kyra Ann Hermann

*Dedicated to my family, that they
may always know that the infinite wisdom
of healing is within themselves.*

"A hero is one who heals their own wounds
and then shows others how to do the same"
-
Yung Pueblo

Table of Contents

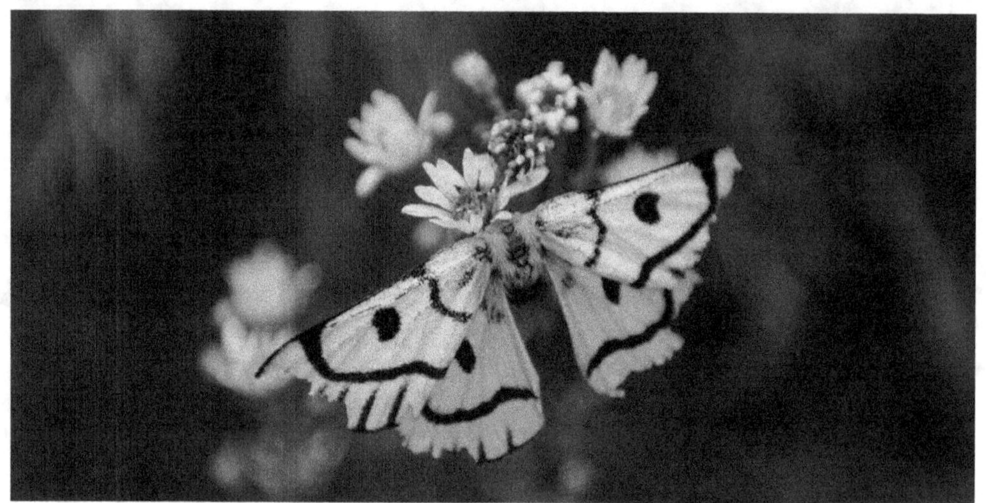

Introduction

The greatest way for me to introduce this book is to introduce you to a vulnerable story about myself. My desire to write this book stems from my journey from a very dark place, to now a place of light, health and learning. My greatest wish is that at least one person can glean a portion of truth that will help them in their journey to reaching optimal health and wellness!

I've always considered myself to be somewhat health conscious. Even as a child I opted for sugar-free whole grain cereals instead of Fruity Pebbles, and I was happy to order myself a salad while my family enjoyed burgers on a weekend out. From a young age I struggled with mystery stomach pains, seemingly brought on by nothing in particular. I was able to manage it for the most part, but the worry of getting sick helped to keep me aware of what I was putting into my body... Unless of course that thing was mac and cheese. I'm quite certain a life without mac and cheese isn't a life at all!

In 2016 I was blessed to give birth to my oldest son, Shilo. Him coming into my life was and is one of the most wonderfully life changing events I've experienced. However, shortly after he was born I began experiencing physical discomforts and mysterious symptoms. It seemed that any foods I ate would leave me feeling sluggish, bloated, and nauseous. I didn't think anything of my condition, believing that this was normal as a tired new mom.

When my Shilo was about 3 months old, I began choking on my food. When I say choking, I mean I struggled to swallow even water without it getting caught in my throat. It felt as if I was trying to swallow through a coffee straw. I spent many nights with food getting impacted in my throat and I would have to force myself to throw up so I could breathe. It was scary as in many of these instances I was home alone. I realized that I needed to get some help.

After getting testing done with my primary care physician and a gastroenterologist, it was determined that I had a diagnosis of "Eosinophilic Esophagitis" (also known as EoE). This condition is an autoimmune disease that functions similar to asthma, in that there is an influx of eosinophils present, but instead of affecting the respiratory tract, it causes restriction of the esophagus. I was sent home with a prescription and no other answers, or hope. The prescription was one that I had consequently already been taking on and off through my life to treat my stomach pains. Because of this, the only known treatment of my illness wasn't effective. I was told I would be submitted to bi-monthly physical stretching of my esophagus, steroidal therapy, and a lifetime of dealing with the ills of my diagnosis.

The first couple of weeks after my diagnosis I allowed myself to be a victim. I sat around, feeling sorry for myself…. Thinking about how it wasn't fair and that everyone else around me could eat and do whatever they wanted without repercussion. From that point, I continued to get more sick. I was reacting to almost every food, causing my EoE to flare up and rendering me unable to eat and swallow. I started to experience horrible bloating 24/7, a stomach distension that would have led an onlooker to believe I was 7 months pregnant.

I quickly realized that I could not live my life like this. I utterly refused to believe that I was doomed to live with a chronic condition that didn't even allow me to have the basic human comforts of eating and existing without pain. I decided to start paying attention to the foods I was eating since I could see there was some connection between the inflammation I was experiencing and what I was putting into my body. I tried my best to eat what was "healthy", buying packaged foods that said they were "natural" and avoiding what I thought could be my trigger foods. I tried multiple fad diets seeking in desperation for relief. But, my health continued to decline.

I decided to see a naturopathic physician in my area, hoping to find answers from a naturally minded practitioner. I got biomeridian testing (also called electro-dermal testing), which is essentially a machine that measures resistance along different acupressure points and electric/energetic pathways (meridians) in the body. This can help to determine if the body is experiencing any kind of inflammation from things such as toxins, pathogens, food sensitivities, nutritional deficiencies, stressors, and weakness or imbalances in different organs of the body. After getting my testing done, I came up with 7 different food sensitivities, the presence of parasites, weakness in all of my organs, heavy metal toxicity, and more. I was given about 5 different homeopathic remedies along with several different supplements and some packets on anxiety. I felt even more lost and confused than I did before! My naturopath did all he could to help me and give me answers. But I just felt like my body was falling apart, that it was betraying me, and I had absolutely no control over my life.

From this point I started falling into a downward spiral. I tried following the recommendations from my doctor as well as buying into different diet plans from people online to try to get answers about my body. I did everything I could to find someone who could give me all the answers. I lost an incredible amount of weight, as an already petite person I dwindled down to about 89 lbs during my worst moments. I started having tingling in my nerves, aching joints, hair loss, fatigue,hormone imbalances, thyroid malfunction, migraines, anxiety attacks and depression. I acted like everything was fine when I was around everyone else, but deep inside I really lost touch with who I was. I started hyper-focusing on my diet, which was the only thing I felt like I was in control of at the time. I became so obsessed that I would only eat avocados and vegetable smoothies and I slowly developed symptoms of an eating disorder called Orthorexia. Orthorexia is usually characterized by someone who becomes obsessed with eating healthy and over-restricts foods. Anxiety, distancing from family/friends, strict control over eating, and irrational fear usually accompany this kind of disordered eating. Listening to all the different health fads gave me so much anxiety about what to eat or what to do. I felt like everything I did could hurt me or make me more sick. I kept trying different one-size-fits all approaches to my health and came up unsuccessful.

My "rock bottom" came one unsuspecting evening. I had started to have an autoimmune flare up again and it just made me so angry. I was angry that I was doing everything I could to eat healthy and be perfect but it didn't feel like it was working. I started sobbing on my bedroom floor with my face pressed into the carpet. I was sobbing in big, ugly gasps that started to turn into hyperventilating. I couldn't breathe and all in a big flurry my son started screaming in the other room. As I started crawling down the hallway my vision was blurring and my hands were curling up to my chest. I army crawled to the living room and started calling 911. I felt my whole body become paralyzed and I layed on the floor next to the phone trying to answer the questions of the first responder on the other end. My speech started slurring and I could feel myself passing out. Shortly after that the paramedics arrived and put me on oxygen. I remember thinking I was having a stroke, or a heart attack, or something terrible! After I started to regain consciousness and my body relaxed I was informed that I had had a panic attack. I laughed because the whole time they were there I kept telling them "thank you for saving me from my stroke!" haha. As hard as that time was it was also mildly amusing because at that point I was still pretty un-aware of the fact that I was struggling with anxiety. I had literally gotten so anxious that my body just shut down. That night left a pretty big imprint on me, and I realized that something needed to change. I was also a little disappointed that I didn't have bragging rights for at least surviving a heart attack... but something tells me that is for the best.

I wish I could say that things got better overnight, but they didn't right away. I started to recognize that the approach I was taking had something fundamentally wrong with it. I was running from doctor to doctor, to instagram influencer, and even to essential oils ladies to ask for them to give me all the answers. I was hyper-focusing on my "diagnosis" and on only one very small part of my overall health. I had become very unbalanced, and was neglecting my mental/emotional and spiritual selves, especially my intuitive self. In that moment I realized that I needed to turn to a power greater than myself. I grew up christian and have always had a firm belief in God. I started praying for guidance and asking for help to know what path to take to best help myself. I felt a lot of strength, guidance and intuition come into me at that point in my journey. I started journaling and trying to be keenly aware of the life events, foods, supplements, exercise, etc that impacted me (for better or for worse). I focused on eating a balanced and healthful diet while also being mindful of foods I knew were not nourishing my body or causing me reactions. I used spiritual guidance, research, and intuition to help me to determine how to approach my specific deficiencies and health concerns. Most importantly I realized that our society has a culture that leads us to believe that doctors know our bodies better than we do. We have completely lost touch with the idea that we have the power to understand the needs of OUR OWN body, especially with spiritual guidance. No one has all the answers for our health. Once I understood that it was up to me to take control of my own health and find the answers for myself, I started to see much better results. I was no longer a victim of my diagnosis, doomed to a lifetime of being told what to do to stay alive.

After 3 months of following the impressions I received about what to learn and study so I knew what to do for myself, I started to see vast improvements. I tried to focus on listening to my body and being willing to try things that I was attracted to. I used food as medicine for my body, and nourished my spiritual and mental/emotional self as well. Holistic healing includes balancing and healing of the whole body, not only the physical.

I was well and thriving for a few months until getting pregnant again with my second son. I enjoyed a healthy pregnancy with all the same woes of diarrhea, aches, and cravings most pregnant women experience. I was blessed with a healthy birth and have been in good health since that time. I will be honest and say that my journey isn't over and I definitely haven't arrived. I am still regularly dealing with small digestive upsets, and trying to manage my anxiety. But I'm not here sharing a story about being "cured" and in 100% perfect condition. I don't think we ever reach perfection in this life. I am here however to share a story of hope. I believe that the body can and does heal. With the help of God (the universe, Spirit, mother earth, or whatever you believe in), and the plants we are provided on the earth I know we can experience healing, abundance, health and wellness. Every day I learn more about nourishing my body/spirit and every day I feel more in tune with the wellness and peace within myself. That is a gift I want to share with everyone I meet. You are the captain of your own ship, and you choose the course.

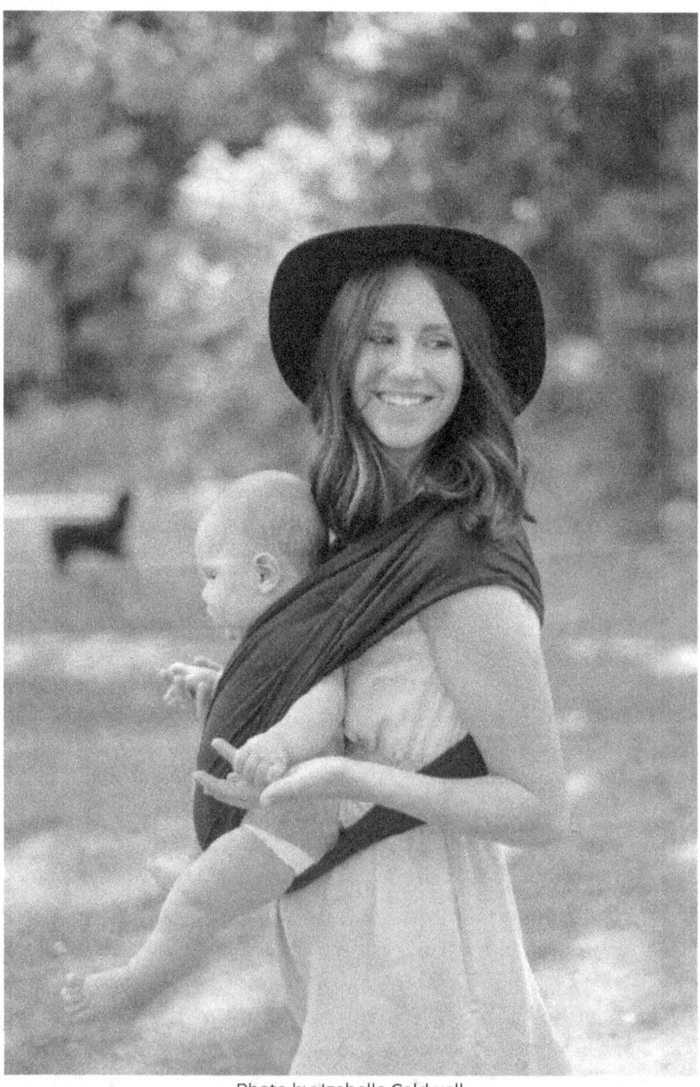

Photo by: Izabelle Caldwell

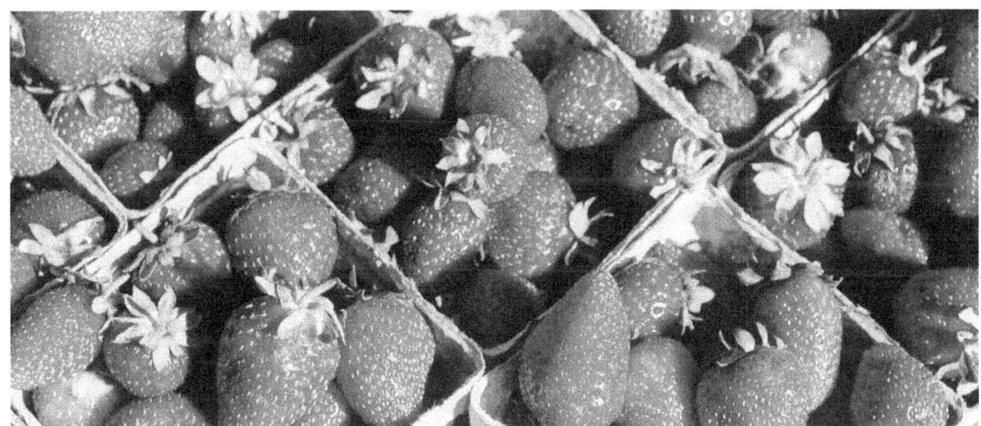

The Medicinal Power of Food

"Let food be thy medicine, and medicine be thy food"
- Hippocrates, The Father of Medicine

Now that you know a little bit of background on me, I'd love to share how my philosophy has changed and adapted over time in regards to how to nourish my body. Although my beliefs about health include taking a balanced holistic approach, in this book we will focus on the physical. I started out believing food and what you eat didn't really impact you, along with most of the population including much of the medical community. Then, because of my experiences I morphed into thinking food was going to hurt me. Along the way I've gotten caught up in many of the trends and fad dieting from counting calories/macros to avoiding carbs, and everything in between. From those extremes, I've now settled into a sustainable and healthy lifestyle that has brought me a lot of happiness. Because of the intense healing I've experienced, I want to share with you what has worked for me.

This isn't a book meant to share with you the "cure all" or "miracle diet". I don't believe in a one-size-fits-all to health. Anyone who says that their way is the only way of healing or the only way of healthy living is someone to be suspicious of. The fact of the matter is, I can't write a book about what is going to work perfectly for you because that is going to be different for every single one of you. Your doctor, your nutritionist, your mom, your husband, or the internet cannot tell you what the right thing is to do for your body. The only people who know that are YOU and your higher power.

I do believe that foods, plant foods and herbs in particular, have very powerful medicinal qualities. I have seen that effect in my own life and in the lives of hundreds of people I have met, worked with, and read about. When you understand the body and how it uses nutrients as tools to rebuild and regenerate, as well as the fact that plants and herbs provide these exact tools/nutrients... You can see a reciprocal and symbiotic relationship between food, the body and it's healing process. The more you open your mind to the medicinal power of food, the more you will be led to using them for your utmost nourishment.

EATING INTUITIVELY

One of the best decisions I made for my health was learning to eat intuitively. Eating intuitively means that you have an instinctual and keen understanding of how your body relays messages to you about what your nutritional needs are, and how to meet them. It also helps to have a little basic understanding about foods, what foods are healthy, etc. which I will share a bit about later in the book.

The reason why I am such a firm believer in intuitive eating is because our body is extremely smart. At our core we have basic instincts for survival. Our culture and the way our society is now has bred a lot of our instincts out of us, and as a whole we are very out of touch intuitively. Our ancestors for example, didn't have the government giving them a food pyramid detailing what was expected of them to eat and in what portions or advertisements manipulating them into believing lies about food. They simply used their instincts to eat what was around them in the portions and combinations that they learned over time were nourishing to their bodies. That is something that we are all completely capable of doing. But this knowledge and connection doesn't come overnight.

Often when I begin to teach someone about intuitive eating, they start by telling me "well, I crave Arby's sandwiches at lunch and ice cream at night... That must be what my body needs!" The trickiest part of learning this way of eating is to learn to distinguish between a craving and a need for nourishment. There are many reasons why we crave food: emotional needs, stress, the presence of pathogens, being overly hungry, low in energy, nutrient deficient, bored, or trying to numb from life in general are a few examples. My general rule when determining if it is a craving or a need is asking myself:

"will this food nourish my body in a healthy way?"

if the answer is yes: go for it!

If the answer is no: don't disregard it.

Ask yourself more questions to understand the source of the craving.

"Am I under a lot of stress? Do I need comfort? Am I bored?".

If you can answer yes to these questions, then it is still okay to meet the craving, but try to consider an "upgrade" that can still meet the emotional need while also providing nutritional nourishment. A great personal example is, I always crave sweets at night. I often opt for apples dipped in homemade chocolate hazelnut spread over binging on candy, or coconut nicecream instead of eating a tub of rocky road (see recipes)

Another important thing to note about cravings is that sometimes it is an indication of a deficiency within the body and your body is asking for that nutrient within the realm of foods you are aware of. For example, if you are craving an Arby's sandwich you may find that you are needing more iron (red meat contains sufficient levels of iron). Or if you always begin craving sugar around 2pm, you are likely low in energy and your body is asking for carbohydrates (the main source of energy from food). It is in these situations that it would benefit you to know a little about food so that you can find some healthier alternatives. You could easily find the iron you need in a large green smoothie with lots of spinach or maybe a small grass-fed steak if you consume meat. The sugar you're craving could be curbed by a food providing a boost of energy such as a bowl of fruit (healthy carbohydrates) or even a satiating source of energy from fat like an avocado or a handful of nuts.

Be gentle with yourself through this process and remember that it is more damaging to criticize yourself for what you're eating than it is to make a lot of mistakes along the way, but ultimately learning to read the needs of your body.

Another important aspect in my journey to learning to intuitively eat is food journaling. Journaling is a great way to document how you respond to certain foods. This response can be emotional, physical, or mental. Either way, it helps to capture a picture of what is making you thrive, and what isn't.

How I have approached it is by simply keeping a notepad on my countertop. At each meal I will think about what I feel like eating. I'll ask myself some questions to determine if what I'm feeling is intuitive or a craving. I'll do my best at that point to eat what I have available, and then I'll write it down. Throughout the day, if I have any feelings or symptoms I will write those too! Some examples could be "2pm I am feeling very low in energy" or "10am I feel really good about myself". I've also written things like "30 minutes later, I am feeling very bloated", "I am constipated, or had diarrhea" , "I had heartburn over the weekend", "I felt anxious/depressed 2 hours later" or "I had a lot of extra energy during my workouts". This type of documentation will help you to draw parallels between how your eating affects your whole body. If you don't believe that food really affects you - then why not experiment for yourself?

I would recommend trying to food journal for at least 6 weeks. During this time, there doesn't need to be any strictness. Feel free to experiment and play. Make note of useful observations and patterns that you notice. If you're seeing that your usual hamburger dinners at night are making you bloat or feel sluggish the next day, try changing that meal to see the effects. If you recognize that you are dealing with a degree of inflammation in connection to the consumption of certain foods, consider removing them for a time to see how you feel.

The reason why I recommend food journaling for a minimum of 6 weeks is because often times reactions or responses to food are not immediate. For example, if you do notice a sensitivity to a food and decide to remove it, you won't see an improvement for around 2-3 weeks because that is how long it takes for that food to fully leave your body/bloodstream. It can also be that it takes awhile to see how eating affects your overall well being mentally and spiritually. It is worth it to take a studious period to learn about yourself and get in touch with your body so that you can enjoy a lifetime of being able to know what you need with little effort.

After those 6 weeks, try listing all your observations and painting a picture for yourself about what you've learned about your body. Using what you've learned, make goals to implement changes. Put those changes into action and continue to journal about how those changes affect you. It took me about 3 months of regular food journaling to understand a lot about the foods that were nourishing me, and ones that were not. I have fine-tuned over time, but those first diligent months completely changed the way I was able to perceive food and enabled me to really make positive decisions for my health.

I recognize there are many things that go into developing the way we approach food: upbringing, religious convictions, ethics, compassion for animals, emotional needs, and our taste buds! Try to be open minded and let go of these preconceived notions during the journaling period. I began my food journaling after having been a vegan for several months. It was difficult for me to let go of my ideologies I had formed for ethical and compassionate reasons, but I experimented with animal products for a long time so I could know I was truly eating intuitively. I now have returned to a very similar way of eating but with the flexibility I need to eat intuitively, and I am thriving well this way. This is an example of what you may experience. You may also eat a lot of a certain food, such as breads and cheeses and find in this process that they are not productive foods for your body, or maybe they are. Be willing to let go, be open, and adapt. Also remember to ask for help and guidance from your higher power in this process. I know you will find great success.

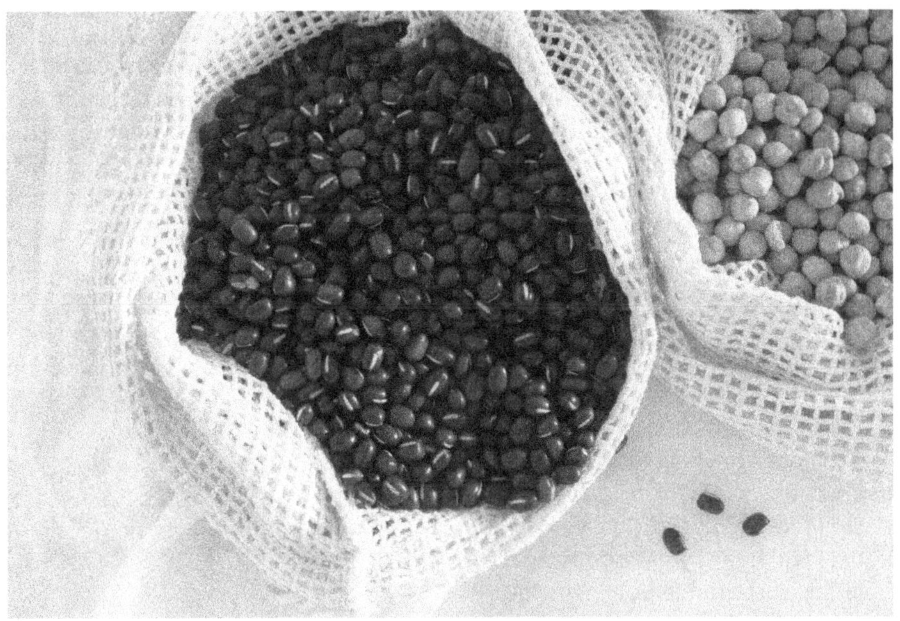

WHAT IS THE PERFECT DIET?

One of the most soul-wrenching questions I have ever wrestled with is, "what is the perfect diet?". I am convinced that when I die, that is the very first question I will ask God…. That and maybe if the dress is blue and black or white and gold. From my teen years I can solemnly say I have tried about every single fad diet or cleanse available. Not necessarily out of a search for weight loss but actually in the search of understanding what is truly healthy. I've had moments of for sure thinking I had the ONLY way to health completely understood…. Only to read a study a week later and feel like my whole foundation was crumbled. I've also failed miserably at multiple dieting attempts. My families personal favorite was when I was 16 and decided I was a staunch vegetarian. I refused meat at the dinner table and made sure everyone knew an animal would not be harmed by my accord. About a week into it, we went out to a buffet for dinner. My sister glanced casually over to my plate, only to audibly (to my family's delight) inform me that my bacon "was not vegetarian". We enjoyed a good laugh as I gasped and admitted to completely forgetting. Lets just say I didn't revisit my vegetarian ways for a long time because I was certain I couldn't live without bacon if it was in fact meat. We live in such a confusing world of differing opinions, contradicting facts, and tried and true testimonials.

I'm going to add another opinion to this sea of opinions and say this: there IS NO perfect diet for everyone. I truly believe that. There are so many factors that go into each person: genetics, epigenetics, where you live, accessibility to food, how you were raised, exposure to certain environmental toxins, different health conditions, emotional state, body type, gender, spiritual convictions, exposure to pathogens, gut health, predisposition to inflammation, personal preferences, and more! Because of this, I believe the "perfect diet" is the one you intuitively create for yourself based on the needs of your body.

There are a few guidelines that I have used to help me to determine if the way I am eating is the best for my body, that I'll share with you! I usually ask myself these questions:

1. Is the way I'm eating high in nutrients?
2. Is the way I'm eating nourishing my body properly?
3. Am I eating whole foods, in their original form?
4. Does this way of eating align with my moral/spiritual values?
5. Do I feel happy eating this way?
6. Do I feel healthy eating this way?
7. Is this sustainable as a lifestyle?
8. Am I following my own intuition, or what someone else says?

As long as I can answer positively to these questions, I feel comfortable with what I am doing. I think it is important that each person identify what lifestyle eating habits help them to feel positive when they answer these questions. If you are in a place where you simply can't answer these questions, then I hope that this book will help give you a place to start in your journey of understanding your relationship to food.

It's okay to enjoy learning everything you can about the "keto diet" or about how to eat certain macros to reach your fitness goals - but at the end of the day, make sure that you have centered yourself and brought it back to checking that knowledge with your intuitive self to see where that fits in.

It is also important that you don't restrict yourself. You should never feel deprived. Try to avoid thoughts and behaviors that seek to "punish" you for overeating or eating poorly, or to stop eating. This is very damaging and will lead to disordered eating. You also want to be mindful of over-eating. I use a simple mantra to help me decide how to approach my portion sizes. "Eat when you are hungry, and stop when you are full". It's that simple! Slowly chewing each bite, staying focused on eating (not being distracted with your phone/tv), and giving yourself space to digest can help significantly! If you have a bad day and eat 5 bowls of popcorn at 10pm like I often find myself doing... Just accept yourself and move on. Try again the next day! It takes practice, but before you know it you will be able to intuitively guide yourself in a healthy way that brings you happiness.

BUT WHAT ABOUT WEIGHT LOSS?

Our society's concentration on and worry about weight loss has completely robbed us of understanding genuine health. We have come to believe that to be healthy you have to be skinny. That you have to have a bikini body or big arms. But I will tell you right now that your body composition can and usually does have very little to do with your actual state of health.

Being healthy has much more to do with how you feel, than how you look. It has more to do with how you are nourishing your body with nutrients, than how many calories you are consuming. Calories are indicative of energy in vs energy out. That is important in some regard, yes. But it should not be the focus. Let me share with you an example: it is very possible for someone to consume strictly white minute rice and tilapia fish ONLY, every single day for years and they might look like they have a great body. But these people are not NOURISHED. If you ask them, they are often struggling with constipation, hormone imbalances, acne or other skin issues, bloating, or overall discontented with the way they feel. Most of the time they are even discontented with they way they look. Why is that? That is because they are not nourishing their body. They are not giving their body the tools that it needs to regenerate, to heal, to build, and to thrive. This pattern of living is unhealthy and it is also not sustainable. Eating this way to have a perfectly lean body will not last for the rest of your life. If you have a goal to meet for a short time and feel intuitively that this is your path - then I support you! But do not be fooled into a cycle of unhealthy eating habits, poor body image, and the absence of true wellness.

I have always believed that if you eat right for your body, you will naturally fall into a healthy weight for you. I will add to this that it is necessary that you are actually eating healthfully, and truly asking yourself the questions we talked about earlier in this chapter. Let me also talk about "a healthy weight". A healthy weight might not be what the movie stars look like. It might not include a 6 pack (although, it could!). Each person has a median weight that is healthy for them, and that can't be determined by any chart, fitness coach, or doctor. That can only be determined by you. Having womanly curves, a little belly, some fat at your thighs, under your arms and in your cheeks is in many cases very healthy. Your natural weight will be very different from those around you. I personally never weigh myself, and I haven't known my weight for over a year. I don't care what I weigh because I know I am sitting at my natural weight and nourishing my body properly.

An even bigger portion of weight loss that has nothing to do with eating habits or exercise is your emotional and mental well being. No matter what you eat or do, if you do not love yourself and are not in tune with your body, you will not be satisfied with the way it looks. As an example, my 16 year old self would have been thrilled to be 95lbs. But when I was ACTUALLY 95 lbs... I still hated my body, because at my core I didn't love myself. A year and a half later, I totally loved my body at 50 lbs heavier and 9 months pregnant, when I was emotionally healthy. It is SO important that you understand that to be in a truly healthy state you must love and accept yourself where you are now. Just because you are loving and accepting yourself doesn't mean you need to stay the same, if you have desires to improve your health or body shape. It just means that you are okay with YOU on a deep emotional level. If you are not okay with you, this process will be very difficult. It will be difficult because the very essence of eating and living healthfully lies within connecting to and accepting what is divinely within you already. If you are living in a constant state of running from yourself, seeking to change everything about yourself, and disliking who you are and what you see in the mirror then it is very hard to accept your intuition.

That doesn't mean that it's impossible. This just means that right now in this moment, you need to take on a self-awareness. Be aware of your habit of seeking the "answers" for happiness from other places. Realize that the answers to your happiness are already within yourself.

UNDERSTANDING HOW FOOD AFFECTS THE BODY

Now that we have worked to become intune with the body, and tried to let go of unhealthy thought patterns surrounding food - it is also important to understand what foods will actually nourish you!

My philosophy about foods that nourish you is very simple. I believe that foods that nourish you are whole foods, in their original form. Well, what does that mean? Whole foods are foods that have not been changed, processed, added to, or taken away from. Let me give you an example. Let's discuss the humble potato. A potato, in its whole form, would be freshly rooted out of the ground. It might even have a little dirt on it! Now, it would be a little unreasonable at this point to take a bite out of the potato and call it dinner. But if you rinse it, cut it up and steam it, then maybe even mash it... It becomes something that many of us enjoy as a comfort food! On the other side of the spectrum, you can drive into the McDonalds drive-thru and order yourself a sizeable helping of french fries. This would not be considered a whole food... For reasons I'm sure you know but I will still explain. When you turn a potato into a french fry, you skin it which strips it of its fiber. You then cut it up and add chemicals and preservatives to it. You then put it in a basket and deep fat fry it in oils that do not exist in nature, and add an inordinate amount of isolated salt (not in its whole form) on top for good measure. This food has been changed, processed, added to and taken away from. The humble potato is no longer a whole food.

I don't want you to believe that eating whole foods means that you can't enjoy them or be creative and flavorful in their preparation! That is quite the opposite.

Going along with our potato example, one of my favorite ways to prepare mashed potatoes is by adding some almond milk, nutritional yeast, sea salt, black pepper, fresh crushed garlic, and serving it with a creamy plant based gravy sauce and mushrooms on top. It is absolutely delicious, while maintaining the integrity and nutrients of the food. If you are a McDonalds french fry addict and wondering how you'll cope with your withdrawals - you will be pleased to know that you can even make fries in a way that will better maintain the nutrients that the potato has to offer without any negative effect to your body. You'll see a recipe for that later in my book.

When you eat something, it can have one of three effects: it will nourish your body, it will be unproductive, or it will cause inflammation to your body. You will eat roughly 85,000 meals in your life. These meals will directly affect the outcome of the health of your body. Do you want that effect to be nourishing, unproductive, or damaging? It is up to you!

NOURISHING VS UNPRODUCTIVE FOODS

When it comes to determining the foods that will nourish your body, it is pretty simple. There are no secret or magical foods. They are foods that have been around for thousands of years, maybe even millions. If you are looking to provide your body with the best possible nutrients, basing your eating habits on the following nourishing foods:

1. Fruits

Fruits are some of the most nutrient dense foods on the planet. They are high in a variety of vitamins, minerals, and antioxidants that are absolutely necessary for healing and optimal health. Fruits naturally and powerfully boost the immune system. There are hundreds of varieties of fruit out there. You can either enjoy eating as many as you can for a variety of nutrients, or you can try eating local fruits in season as that too has its own benefit. Now matter how you slice it, you need to eat fruit every single day. Don't believe the fad that fruit sugar is somehow bad for you, or that they are too high in "carbs". The fiber present in fruit helps to balance the natural fructose. Fruit is one of the most nourishing foods you can give your body. For best results, eat fruit first thing in the morning to support your body's natural detox. Eating fruit alone instead of mixed into a meal, or 15 minutes before your meal is also beneficial as fruit digests more quickly than other foods.

2. Vegetables

Along with fruits, vegetables are also immensely dense with important nutrients. From leafy greens to grounding root vegetables, vegetables provide us with chlorophyll, antioxidants, fatty acids, vitamins, minerals, and serve as a powerful source of plant energy. Often seen as a humble "side" in the form of canned green beans or corn, vegetables flavor and versatility can go unappreciated. Aim to eat leafy greens, and a variety of other vegetables every day, multiple times a day. Many vegetables are a surprisingly good source of protein. Not only are vegetables filling, but they are very healing for the body. Try to buy local and organic when possible, as the nutrient content of the vegetable will depend on the soil it grows in. If you struggle with keeping produce from going bad, consider buying vegetables (and fruits) frozen. They still retain their nutrients in this way. Just make sure you never microwave them to thaw them.

3. Beans / Legumes

Beyond their magical flatulent creating capabilities and keeping Taco Bell in business, beans (and legumes) are rich sources of nutrients! High in protein, high in fiber, and also high in minerals, these plants are versatile and delicious additions to a healthy diet. Beans and legumes serve as a great "staple" for many meals including soups, curries, stir fries, salads, casseroles, stews, cultural dishes and more. Combined with certain grains, they become a complete protein and are a great plant source to regenerate muscles for athletes. When sprouted, beans and legumes become especially high in nutrients, boosting the vitamins and minerals as much as 500%. If you don't sprout your beans and legumes, consider soaking them for the best digestibility of the food. Try to enjoy one or more servings of beans and legumes daily! Some examples of beans and legumes are: black beans, pinto beans, chickpeas, lentils, peanuts, peas, and soy.

4. Grains

Although they have recently gotten a bad reputation in the health world, grains have been an essential staple in the human diet for at least 100,000 years. Grains, when eaten in their whole form are high in fiber, vitamin e, b vitamins, several minerals, phytochemicals and healthy fats. Grains are often frowned upon because they have the tendency to cause digestive upsets in sensitive individuals. This is because they are harder to digest due to the presence of certain anti-nutrients. If prepared correctly through soaking, sprouting, fermenting, and low heating methods, grains can often be well tolerated by most individuals. What's more is that grains have evolved to be heavily genetically modified crops, as well as sprayed with pesticides. When choosing grains, make sure that you buy organic, non-gmo varieties and buy them in their whole food form rather than processed. When dealing with a chronic inflammatory health condition, it is wise to consider taking a break from grains during the healing process if they give you trouble. Otherwise, grains are a healthy and delicious addition to a balanced diet. I usually enjoy 1-2 servings of grains daily. Some examples are: whole wheat, oats, wild rice and other varieties, buckwheat, millet, amaranth, barley, rye, and quinoa (also considered a seed).

5. Nuts / Seeds

Nuts and seeds are a delicious source of healthy fat and protein. Many of them contain healthy omega-3 fatty acids which support health brain function. They are versatile savory snacks, bringing flavor and texture to any meal they are added to. When choosing nuts and seeds, remember to avoid roasted and salted varieties. These are considered processed and often lack their original nutrients. Buy your nuts and seeds raw in bulk and if you wish, low heat them with your own spices or add them the granolas, salads, butters, milks, sauces, and more. You will find many recipes in this book that take advantage of the versatility of nuts and seeds as well as their supreme nutrition. Some examples of nuts and seeds are: almonds, cashews, walnuts, hazelnuts, macadamia, pistachio, sunflower seeds, pumpkin seeds, hemp, chia, and flax.

6. Herbs and Spices

Herbs and spices are extremely medicinal in nature. For such small and unnoticeable plants, they pack a nutritional punch. Herbs can be used to powerfully heal any ailment of the body, whether it is communicable illness or chronic disease. Herbs are best used every day, in sizeable portions over a period of time. This is especially true if you are hoping to see their healing benefits. Even if you are already in good health, it is beneficial to use herbs in each meal as spices or a flavorful garnish. Teas and tinctures are also great ways to ingest herbs. You can also add them to fresh green juices or smoothies to boost their nutrients and detoxifying effects. Some examples of herbs are: ginger, turmeric, basil, cilantro, parsley, cacao, red raspberry leaf, oregano, garlic, vanilla, cinnamon, black pepper, peppermint, and lemon balm.

Try your best to buy produce that is organic, and in the best case from a local farmer who doesn't use irradiation practices. Buying produce in season also helps to ensure the nutrient content of your food as well. If you eat animal products, ALWAYS buy organic from a trusted source and make sure that the animals were grass-fed, pasture-raised, wild-caught and not treated with antibiotics, hormones or steroids. It is always best if you know that these animals were treated with kindness as well.

In the very best case, growing your own fruits and vegetables and getting animal products from your own animals is going to be the best health practice. This is not always accessible for everyone - including me! But I am using this knowledge to set it as a goal for the future, and that is what I hope we can all do as well.

Foods that nourish you are whole foods as we have discussed previously, that are prepared in a way that maintain their nutrients. There are certain practices that can kill or denature the nutrients in food. When that happens, the food goes from being nutrient dense, to being more unproductive. Here are 3 common ways you can damage your foods vital nutrients:

1. Processing

Processing food usually includes stripping away a portion of the plant and isolating another part for consumption. An easy example is white flour. Whole grain wheat contains a vitamin rich wheat germ, which, during processing is stripped away, leaving a substance that contains no nutrients. It is further ground down, and added to man made ingredients and chemicals that the body doesn't recognize or know how to process. Like mentioned with the flour, processing usually also includes adding damaging ingredients that are unnatural for the body such as preservatives, dyes, chemicals, and genetically modified ingredients. These additives are KNOWN to cause cancer, inflammation, and disease.

2. Overheating

The vitamins, minerals, proteins, fats, enzymes and bacteria present in food are very heat sensitive. Heating your foods too high will change the food from an organic, living substance to an inorganic, dead substance. This doesn't mean that there is absolutely no nutritional value. It just means that in many cases you lose a lot of the original nutrient content of the food. VItamins and minerals become non absorbable, proteins become denatured, fats become rancid, and enzymes and bacteria will die. Because of this, it is a good practice to be judicial about the foods you choose to heat and to what temperatures. As a general rule, nutrients in food begin to be lost at 118 degrees F. As someone who struggles to eat foods that are not cooked, I can say that I haven't perfected this practice yet but I am trying to mindful of it. That's the best place to start! Consider low heating foods by steaming and baking as these are some of the least destructive methods. Try to avoid any cooking methods that blacken, burn or char your food. This introduces carcinogens into your body. Microwaving is also not recommended.

3. Irradiating

Irradiating of foods is exposing the foods to ionizing radiation, gamma rays, or other similar methods to preserve food or make it safe for packaging. Some examples would be pasteurization of foods which kills the beneficial bacteria and enzymes (think pasteurized milk), canning food, sterilizing, treating it with pesticides, or treating fruits and vegetables to delay the ripening or sprouting process. These processes have been deemed safe by governmental agencies, however, they do damage the nutrient content of the foods we buy in our grocery stores and store in our pantries.

Processing, heating and irradiating foods can often render them unproductive. That doesn't always make them damaging or bad, nor does it mean you should never consume them. It only means you should be aware that if a large part of your diet, or all of your diet is affected by these processes, you are likely consuming a mostly unproductive diet nutritionally.

Processed foods are also unproductive. Its best to to practice avoiding processed foods altogether. Even the processed foods you see that label themselves as "healthy" or that you find in the health food store are not nourishing for your body. Skip the packaged foods also, and consider buying things like grains, beans/legumes, nuts and seeds in bulk and storing them yourself. This is also another way to ensure the nutrients are better than they would be if processed or canned otherwise. This method also proves to be cheaper and more environmentally friendly.

There are some other practices you can try that will help to increase the nutrient profile of your food. Some examples are fermenting and sprouting your foods! Because I want to give a more in depth description of these practices and teach you how to do them yourself, I have saved for these topics their own chapters that you will find later in the book.

INFLAMMATORY FOODS

Just as foods are very powerful in their ability to nourish our bodies, they are also very powerful in their ability to damage them. Foods can damage our bodies by causing inflammation, depleting other nutrients, introducing toxins, feeding pathogens, introducing things the body cannot absorb, feeding tumors, throwing off body systems, causing build up of mucus or plaque, literally injuring tissues of the body, damaging the gut, and causing chronic illness. Use your intuition to help you navigate how to regulate the presence of these foods in your life. Here are some to be aware of:

1. Sugar

When I say sugar, I am not referring to naturally occuring sugars such as those found in fruit (which are very good!) or others such as raw honey. I am referring to processed sugars such as refined cane sugar, corn syrup and artificial sweeteners. Sugars have been proven to spike blood sugar, cause systemic inflammation, feed pathogens/candida, damage gut health and feed cancers. Artificial sweeteners although they tout health benefits are equally if not more damaging. These man made chemicals cause inflammation in the brain, still cause cancer, and still cause blood sugar problems by confusing the body. Natural sugars such as raw honey, pure maple syrup, dates, and coconut sugar are a much better alternative but are to be used mindfully. Some people are still sensitive to natural sugars, and in this case you can consider other sweeteners such as stevia or monk fruit extract that won't spike blood sugar. Use your intuition.

2. Processed foods

As already discussed, processing strips food of their vital nutrients. Processing also introduces man made chemicals such as preservatives, genetically modified ingredients (gmo's), "natural flavors" (meaning chemicals they aren't required to list), dyes, and foods that have been split, spliced, recombined, and changed so far from their original state that if you think you can't recognize the name on the label - then you can only imagine how much your body doesn't know what to do with them. It is best to avoid processed foods altogether as they can damage your body in every way imaginable.

3. Conventional animal products

Conventional animal products are damaging to the body. If you don't believe this now then this is something I invite you to research immediately. Animals are not only treated inhumanely, being kept in tiny and dirty conditions with disease running rampant, but they are ripped from their families and slaughtered while still alive. The negative emotions, sadness and energy from these animals remains in their bodies and then we consume it. What does this do to our body? As if this isn't enough, these animals are treated with harmful substances such as antibiotics, growth hormones, steroids, and other medications. They also are fed genetically modified corn or soy and even sometimes the remains of other dead and putrefied animals. All of this is retained in the muscles of the animal, and it is absorbed into our bodies when we eat them. I have nothing against the consumption of organic sustainably raised and humanely treated animals, but I do believe that the quality and source of meat is of utmost importance.

4. Dairy products

A noted above, conventional animal products have a damaging effect on the body, but especially dairy. All foods fed to the animal as well as chemicals, hormones, steroids, medications and antibiotics are dumped right into the animals breastmilk. Dairy is also a mucus forming food, meaning that it can cause inflammation and excess mucus in our bodies. This will lead to chronic conditions like sinus congestion, post nasal drip, cough, mucousy stools, etc. Dairy also is hard to digest. It's protein Casein is not easily absorbed by the human body. Because of this, dairy is a very common culprit to digestive issues such as bloating, gas, IBS, constipation, and acid reflux. We see this often especially in infants struggling with colic and reflux, if they are drinking dairy formula or the mom is eating dairy products and transferring to the breastmilk. Pathogens and viruses in the body also feed on dairy. This means you will be more susceptible to getting sick. The sugar in dairy, Lactose, is also very difficult for human bodies to digest. Studies show that anywhere from 75-90 percent of humans are lactose intolerant (depending on race). Because of this, people respond to the food sensitivity in a variety of ways, commonly with skin problems like acne and eczema, or migraines, ADHD, and mental illness have also been responses. Most dairy products have been pasteurized, meaning that the essential enzymes and bacteria present in the milk has been killed, further making them less digestible. Some opt for raw diary, which can be a slightly more appropriate alternative as it still contains bacteria and enzymes. Lastly, dairy is known to cause inflammation to the body, which disease is always a state of chronic inflammation. As a deep lover of mac and cheese, I know it can be difficult to imagine life without cheese. Follow your intuition.

5. GMO foods

Corn, wheat and soy are extremely genetically modified foods. They are mass produced in such a way that they have come so far from the original plant that they are hardly recognized by the body. They are also highly treated with pesticides. You are hard pressed to find these foods truly non-gmo. With this being said, if you do consume them try your best to find organic and non-gmo options, and remember that the whole food versions will always be kinder to your body.
Soy specifically is estrogenic, meaning it can negatively impact our hormones especially if we are sensitive to that. Corn has evolved to being a very high sugar food, used in massive amounts as high fructose corn syrup. It is low in nutrients, making it unproductive at best. Wheat is better eaten when using its ancient grain friends such as rye, spelt or kamut. These are in their more natural forms. When consuming these foods be mindful, and aware they they could likely be a source of

inflammation for you. Consider practices such as fermenting or sprouting to help these foods to be better for the body.

6.   Vegetable oils

Vegetable oils are of particular concern especially because they are so widely used that you will find them in almost anything. If you are eating at a restaurant (even one that is considered healthy) you will find vegetable oils in shocking amounts. They are in almost all processed and packaged foods as well as any baked good. They are even lurking in foods like nut butters, air popped popcorn, freezer foods, and most "healthy" packaged foods you'll see at the health food store. Vegetable oils are not organic or natural substances. They are processed from the plant in a way that makes them extremely unstable. Especially when heated, they easily go rancid, and when ingested introduce free radicals into the body. They also cause an imbalance in our bodies ratio of omega-3 and omega-6 fatty acids. Because of this, inflammation is almost immediate upon ingesting these oils and they shouldn't be consumed under any circumstances. Examples are: Canola oil, vegetable oil, corn oil, soybean oil, peanut oil, sunflower oil, safflower oil or cottonseed oil. If you want to consume oils, consider the healthy alternatives such as: coconut oil, organic extra virgin olive oil, or avocado oil.

7.   Anything that causes YOU inflammation

Because we are so vastly different, you will find that the list of inflammatory foods may be longer or shorter than the one I have provided. Inflammation presents in many forms, but some examples are: digestive problems, body aches, headaches/migraines, skin breakouts (acne), hormone imbalances, blood sugar imbalances, edema, tingling extremities, joint pain, fogginess, mood swings, depression or anxiety. Food journaling and experience will help you to determine that. For some reason I had a 1 year period where chickpeas would give me the runs no matter what! Odd albeit, I waited it out and learned to sprout them then reintroduce them later. Now I gladly enjoy them in my diet. Instead of eating foods that cause you inflammation, or restricting too much... consider taking a break and upgrading these foods to similar but less stress-inducing options while you heal.

8.   Any food that makes you unhappy

I have met many people who feel like in order to be healthy, they need to eat certain foods even if they hate them. That is simply untrue! In fact, I believe that forcing yourself to eat food that you don't like is doing more damage than good. Imagine the episode in The Office where Michael forces Kevin to bite straight into a stalk of raw broccoli, to which he spits it out and says he is "traumatized". If eating healthy makes you feel traumatized, you're doing it wrong! In most cases, you can find a food that has similar benefits and nutrients but that you enjoy. Or you can learn to prepare it in a way that you like. My husband hates raw cauliflower and butternut squash. I personally enjoy these foods, so I have learned to prepare them in ways that he now loves (as you will see in my recipes). From teriyaki cauliflower bites to creamy alfredo sauce he now enjoys this food when the very thought of it used to make him want to dry heave.

This list is not intended to cause any stress or label all these foods as "bad". But rather, it is to bring awareness to the fact that the foods we eat can have a negative impact. Use your best judgement to determine how to approach this issue. You'll know what to do!

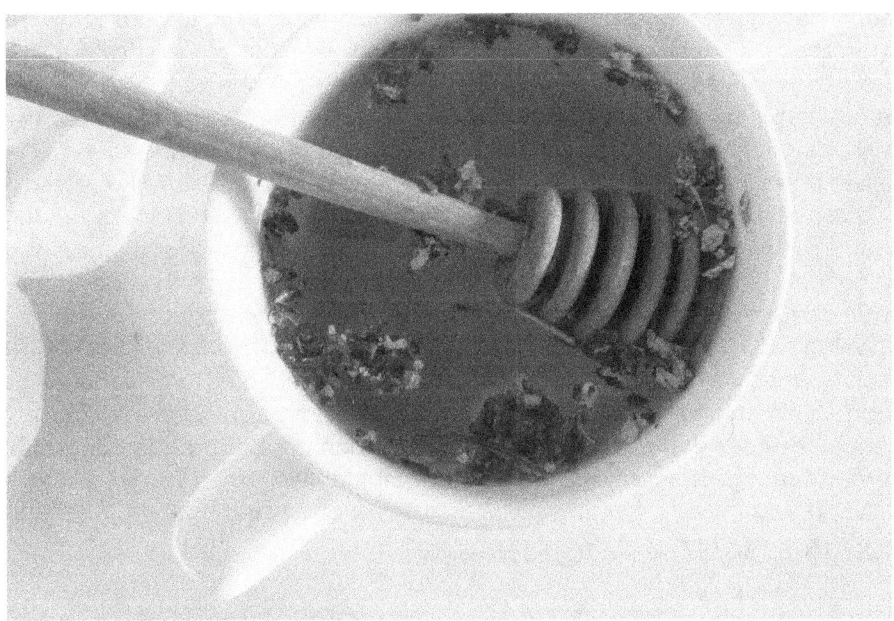

THE MEDICINAL POWER OF FOOD

One of the biggest doubts that people have when I tell them how they can improve their health is that food has any medicinal benefit. I often get comments like "well I grew up on poptarts and kool aid and I'm fine" or, "so and so never eats healthy and they are skinny so I don't see how it makes a difference". One that I find particularly asinine is "I need to let my kids live a little" in regard to giving them fast food and sugar laden foods every day. We have come so far from true health, that we don't even know what it actually looks like! Our definitions of "fine" and "living" are not what it truly means to enjoy a life free of disease and full of the kind of living energy real food provides. Most of the time, the people who believe they are "fine" also fail to mention that they get colds and strep throat several times a year, or they are taking blood pressure and thyroid medications. Even more likely is that they are chronically constipated, and that they think they are fine but won't be fine 10 years from now. Our country is the sickest it has ever been, especially in regard to chronic life long diseases. The leading causes of death in the US are: heart disease, cancer, respiratory disease, alzheimer's, diabetes, influenza and kidney disease. So you tell me - are we fine?

Real, living food and herbs are immensely medicinal. They were created just FOR us, and for our bodies by the supreme creator and the universe. We have subsisted for millions of years on organic plants and animals alone. Ancient groups of people have always used herbs as medicine and quite successfully, to boot.

At their core, food posses the very building blocks we need to survive. Our bodies are comprised of oxygen, hydrogen, vitamins A-Z, minerals, protein/amino-acids, fats, fatty acids, molecules, atoms, bacteria, and enzymes. Food possess all of these in their perfectly absorbable forms. When we consume them, we fuel the body like a perfectly functioning machine to do its work like it was beautifully created to do. Disease occurs when we are starved of these essential building blocks, rendering us unable to heal and regenerate and live happily! Herbs are food for the organs, and foods not only nourish the body but the mind and the soul. When the body does become damaged, it may need help and nourishment to help it get back into functioning order. Herbs and food have the perfect instructions for the body (especially when combined well using intuition and experience) to help it to move in the right direction and overcome these obstacles. I don't believe there is a single ailment in the body that cannot be treated with a bountiful, nutritious, living whole food way of eating. Especially if it is a commitment for life.

HEALING WITH FOOD

There are 2 general approaches to healing. I love these approaches as explained by Dr. John Christopher, a Master herbalist and Naturopathic Doctor. He categorizes the two methods as the "vitalist" approach, and the "atomist" approach.

The vitalist approach is a natural and holistic approach. A vitalist seeks to work WITH the body, and use natural methods of supporting the body in its processes. Vitalists trust in the body and fundamentally believe in its ability to heal on its own when given the right tools. Vitalists also understand that a "symptom" is the way the body communicates that there is something wrong. We do not treat the symptoms, but rather use symptoms as a means to find the "root cause". Vitalists treat the root cause of disease, by healing the body on a cellular level. Food, herbs, and other natural methods support a vitalist approach and is a very successful and long lasting method of healing. Hippocrates, the father of medicine took this vitalistic approach.

An atomist approach seeks to "fix" the body. An atomist at their roots does not believe that the body has the ability to heal on its own, Because of this, they use unnecessary interventions. They also treat the symptoms, instead of the cause. An atomist will intervene with the body by using an unnatural substance to stop a symptom. This intervention-focused approach to healing slows or stops the body from carrying out its own natural healing methods. Western medicine as it is today follows an atomist approach to chronic illness. This leaves the masses taking medications for symptoms, and medications for the side effects of their medications. Unless the root cause is addressed and healed, disease will always abound.

When healing with food, the goal is to take a vitalist approach and work with the body. If you are using foods only to curb a symptom, but not to deal with the root cause, you may find yourself feeling like you're not experiencing the medicinal benefit of food. For example, if you are only eating healthy for a short time, say, to be skinny for your cruise... But then you fall right back into your old eating habits afterward, then you'll not fully benefit from the medicinal qualities in food. The same goes for someone who is feeling ill. I often see people who are only willing to eat well until they feel a little better, and then they will go back to what they were doing before. Using foods medicinally is not a "diet" that you can use short term. It is a lifestyle. If you want to see food transform your life, you will need to commit to eating whole living foods for a long time, ideally for life! The way this works is through daily, constant and concentrated exposure. That is how true, lasting health is built.

Because we live in a world of instant gratification, this concept may be very daunting and difficult to grasp. Don't be dismayed! Although it might not happen overnight, even one small change is a good change and will benefit you immensely. Any step in the right direction is a step in the right direction. I have found that even after 2 years of having this knowledge I am nowhere near perfect. But from where I began at rock bottom to where I am today is a complete 180. You don't have to be chronically ill for this to change your life. I have benefitted physically, mentally and spiritually and my life has been enriched. The instant pleasure of a drive-thru is never as satisfying as a home cooked meal from scratch that nourishes your and your kids bellies. The instant gratification of a weight loss pill is never deeply satisfying like a year or two of diligent healthy eating, exercise and emotional healing. Taking a medication for your entire life and being damaged by its side effects will never bring the joy that living disease free will bring. Even if it's at the expense of your McNuggets and Diet Coke. Choose to work hard now so you can be free later!

If you want to heal with food it is very simple. There is no magical protocol, or mysterious potion. Listen to your body. Eat real whole food. Use herbs daily. Drink lots of pure water. Get good sleep. Nourish your relationships. This, and asking for help and guidance from the higher power you believe in is all it requires. Have faith in the process and love yourself enough to try! You will only find healing.

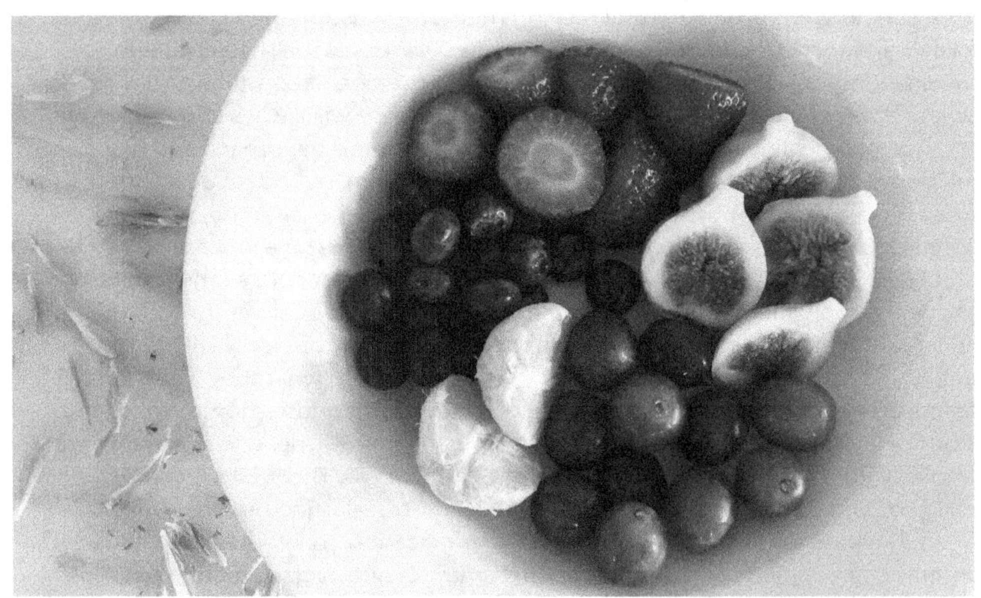

Raw vs Heated foods

"Knowledge is essential to healing"
-Anthony William

Eating foods in their raw form is becoming lost on us as we become more developed as a people. We anciently used to enjoy foods in their raw forms more frequently, but the convenience of microwaves, toasters, ovens, instant fires right on our stove tops and instant pots have lead us to cooking most if not all of our meals. Although there is nothing inherently wrong with this, it does lend itself to us consuming a significantly nutritionally deficient diet.

BENEFITS OF RAW FOODS

Foods in their raw form are considered "living". To make it easy, you know a food is living if you are able to go outside and plant it in the backyard and it will grow a plant, or bring forth a seed. For example, you can plant a grain of whole wheat and it will grow a plant, but if you bury a loaf of bread it won't grow a plant.

Fruits and vegetables freshly picked and untreated contain living enzymes and bacteria on them that increases our ability to digest those foods. These soil based organisms are some of the best probiotics available! They easily make it through the digestion process to the intestines where they nourish your gut and help strengthen your immune system. Raw foods also maintain their highest degree of nutrients in comparison to their cooked friends.

When I speak of "raw" foods I am talking about plant foods, not raw meats. Although some meats are safe consumed raw, because of the handling process the incidence of foodborne illness in raw meats is high and it is preferable that they are cooked before consumption.

Some of the most nutrient dense raw foods available are sprouts, which we will discuss more in depth later in this book. Fruits, vegetables, nuts and seeds can also all be happily consumed in their raw forms.

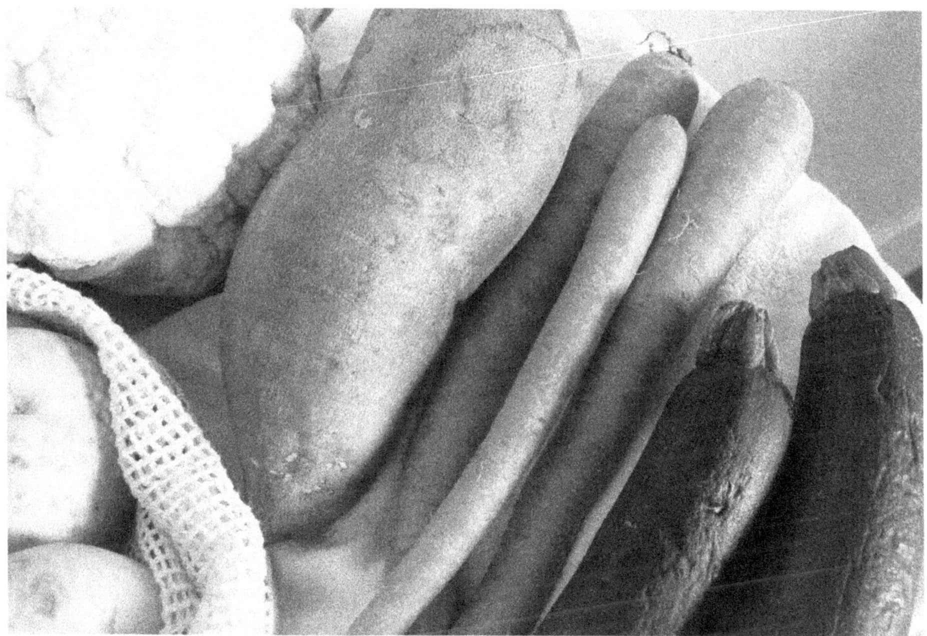

HEATED FOODS

Some foods are more sensitive to damage of nutrients than others upon heating. For example, it is quite difficult to eat root vegetables and some squashes in their raw form so it would be better to them cooked. Potatoes, butternut squash, onions and beets are good examples. Fruit and leafy greens are examples of plants that you want to keep raw when possible!

Plants begin to lose their nutrients starting at 118 degrees fahrenheit This doesn't mean all is lost, but the longer and hotter you cook them, the more you will lose. The presence of water in cooking can also draw out nutrients, as such it is with boiling. Streaming, baking, a light saute or pressure cooking are better ways of heating that help to preserve as many nutrients as possible. It's best to cook only until starting to wilt or aromatic. You don't want your vegetables to be completely black or smooshed. A good one to practice with is zucchini. A light saute for 2 minutes on low heat helps it to be slightly wilted. Much longer and you have a browned mushy mess.

Some sources say microwaving is a good form of nutrient preservation but this simply isn't true. Microwaving is an inorganic way to heat your food and it will damage and change the nutrients so that they are not able to be absorbed by the body. Enough competent material and studies are available on the internet for you to learn the woes of microwave cooking so I won't go into it here, but it sufficeth me to say that you should throw out your microwave if you haven't already.

COOKING WITH OILS

When cooking foods, it is common practice to use oils or animal based fats to help add flavor and ease to cooking. It is important however, to be aware of the different "smoke points" of the oils so that you can make sure you are not heating certain oils too high causing them to go rancid.

Some examples of oils that shouldn't be cooked with are: vegetable oils (which I don't think should be used at all), olive oil and coconut oil. That is because these oils have a smoke point ranging from 200 - 350 degrees F. Once the oils reach their smoke point, they go rancid, emit toxic fumes and contain free radicals. These free radicals are damaging to the body and cause inflammation when ingested. Its best to use olive oil as a salad dressing, and if you do cook with coconut oil make sure it is on a low heat under 350 degrees. Although most of the health benefits of coconut oil are removed once heated anyway.

Oils and fats that contain a higher smoke point are: animal fats like lard, tallow, and ghee (clarified butter), and avocado oil. My personal favorite to cook with is avocado oil, as it's smoke point is 520 degrees F. I also enjoy cooking with ghee when I want a more savory flavor. It is clarified butter, meaning the the milk solids have been removed. This makes it a better alternative for those who are sensitive to dairy.

Some have the opinion that oils in general are considered a processed food and are not a healthy, whole food to consume. I have felt that they provide a healthy amount of fats into my diet so I intuitively enjoy them. Listen to your body to know what is right for you.

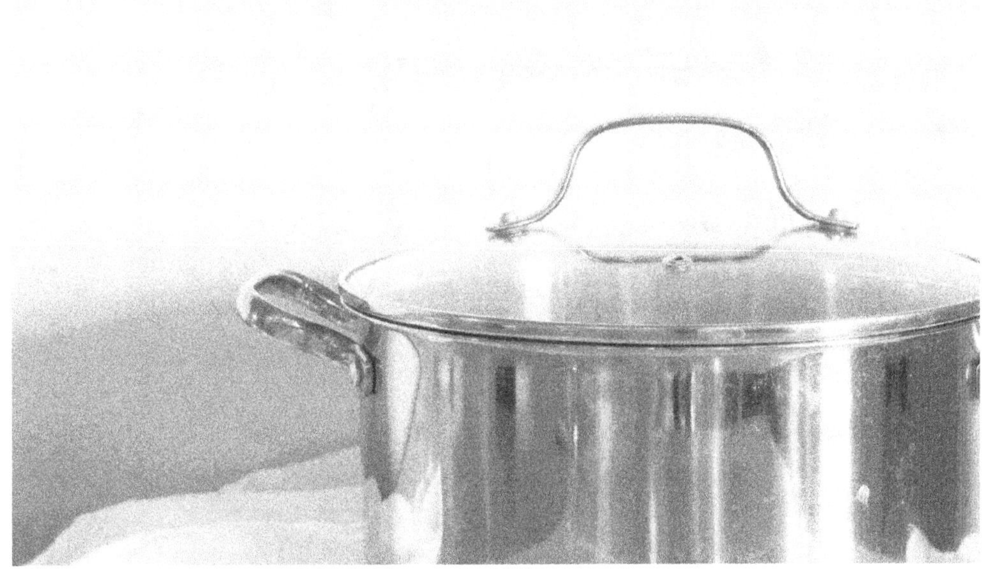

COOKING MATERIALS

Another important aspect to cooking your food is what it is being cooked in. Not all cookware is created equal! Just like everything else, the industry has created high-tech non-stick convenience cookware for the "benefit" of the consumer. These non-stick cookwares contain extremely toxic and carcinogenic chemicals. When you cook your food on these surfaces, the substances get into your food and you ingest them. Some side effects of eating from this type of cookware include developmental delays, inflammation in the brain and neurotoxicity, allergies, thyroid problems, liver toxicity, high cholesterol, and cancer. Be wary of teflon and other non-stick cookware and consider upgrading to a non toxic alternative. Stainless steel, ceramic, cast iron, glass or copper are all good alternatives.

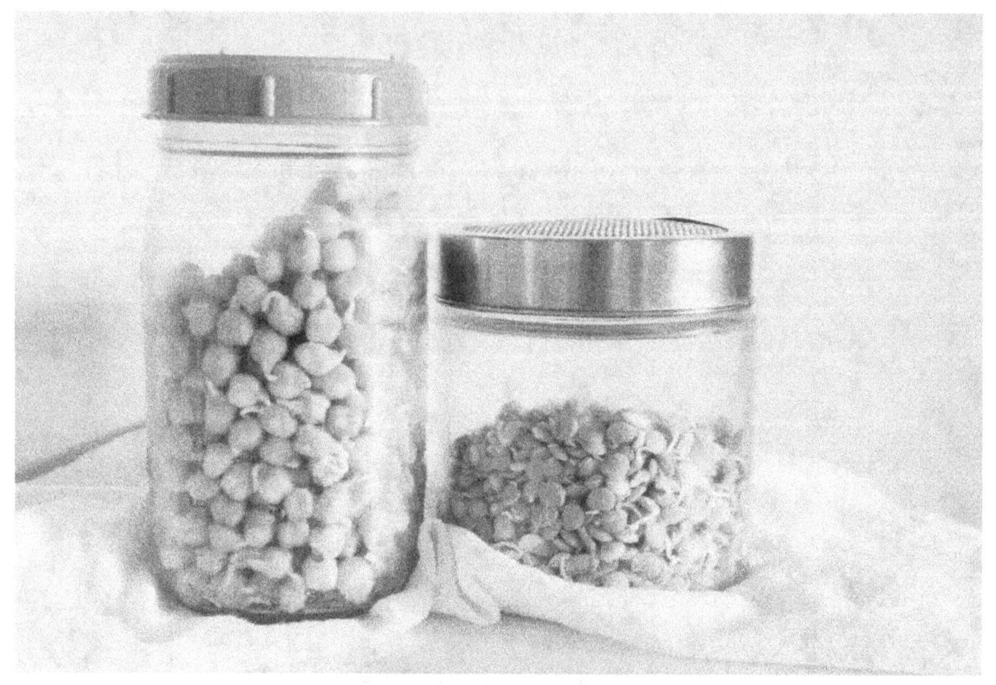

Sprouting

"Don't judge each day by the harvest you reap, but by the seeds that you plant"
-Robert Louis Stevenson

One of the most important aspects of nutrition in my opinion is ensuring that we are nourishing the body as much as possible with vitamins, minerals, enzymes, probiotics, essential fatty acids, proteins and other essential nutrients. A great way to nourish the body is through addition of sprouts to the diet!

WHAT IS SPROUTING?

Sprouting is a natural and simple way of increasing the nutrient profile of your foods as well as improving absorption of said nutrients. A sprout is the beginnings of a plant. You can sprout any seed, nut, grain, or legume by simply soaking it in water, draining, and rinsing it while allowing it to germinate for a period of time (usually around 3-7 days). Not only are you upgrading your food, you are also facilitating the growth of an adorable baby sprout!

BENEFITS OF SPROUTING

- Higher incidence of vitamins and minerals
- Increase in enzymes and probiotics
- Higher levels of essential fatty acids
- More bioavailable nutrients and proteins
- Decrease in and absence of anti-nutrients

Higher incidence of vitamins and minerals

Studies have shown that sprouts contain up to 20 times the amount of vitamin A, B vitamins, Vitamin C and Vitamin E as well as minerals such as selenium, iron, magnesium, calcium, and more. It also boosts the presence of chlorophyll, which is a powerful antioxidant.

Increase in enzymes and probiotics

Enzymes are necessary for all bodily functions. Metabolic enzymes, digestive enzymes, and naturally occuring enzymes found in raw foods are all needed. Sprouts contain up to 100 times more active enzymes than found in their fully grown plant and seed counterparts. Because sprouts are a raw and living food, they are able to offer us a spectrum of living enzymes that will help us to properly digest our foods and therefore increasing nutrient absorption.

Beneficial bacteria is naturally occuring on living organic food (that has not been treated with pesticides), and sprouts are not the exception. Making your own sprouts facilitates the presence of healthy bacteria that will populate your gut and help improve gut health and digestion. Beneficial bacteria also are responsible for important functions such as creating vitamin b12 in the ileum (a part of your intestinal tract). Raw foods are one of natures probiotics!

Higher levels of essential fatty acids

Sprouts have been found to contain up to 30 times more essential fatty acids than the original plant or seed. These fatty acids are helpful for supplying energy to the body, transporting oxygen, and several other functions including acting as anti-inflammatories and containing anti-cancerous properties.

More bioavailable nutrients and proteins

As the sprouting process develops, certain minerals bind to proteins which make them more easily absorbed by the body. Bioavailable nutrients means that the body not only accepts the nutrients into the body, but assimilates them.

Decrease in and absence of anti-nutrients

Anti-nutrients are natural compounds in a plant that are in place to help it protect itself. These compounds interfere with the absorption of nutrients and can be inflammatory to our gut and body. The process of soaking and sprouting breaks down and eliminates the presence of some anti-nutrients. Examples of anti-nutrients are lectins, phytic acid, and gluten.

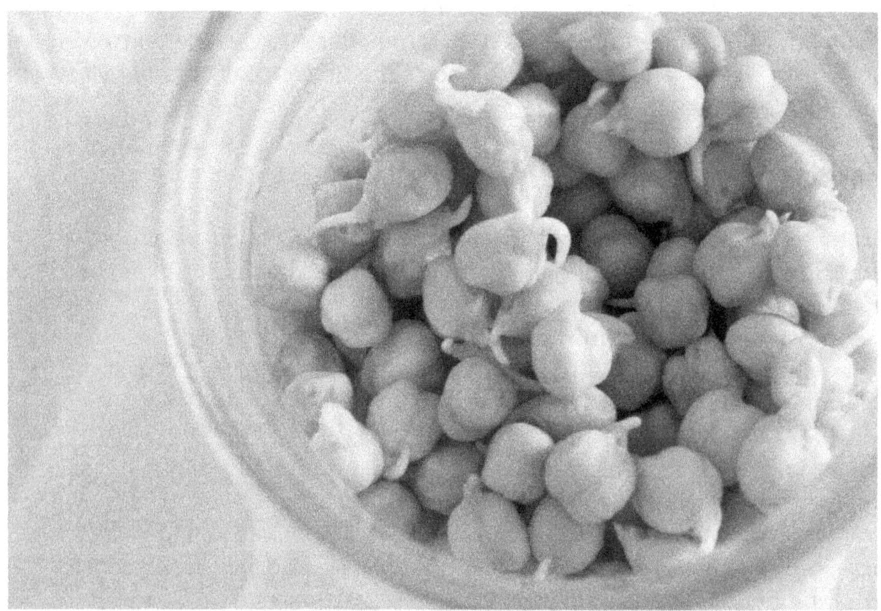

HOW TO SPROUT

How to properly sprout can vary greatly between different plants. Most of them require similar care. Practice or experience will help you to determine how to reap the desired outcome! Here is a simple break down of how to sprout, as well as the tools you'll need.

Tools

- ☐ A sprouting jar with a mesh lid OR a sprouting lid and mason jar
- ☐ Something to prop your jar in. A heavy bowl will do the trick.

<u>Ingredients</u>

- ☐ Your seed, nut, legume or grain of choice
- ☐ Filtered water

<u>Conditions</u>

- ☐ A dark, room temperature area to place your sprouts
- ☐ Love and care from you!

What to do

1. Take your desired amount of seeds, nut, legume or grain (usually around ¼ c - 2 c) and rinse/sort them.
2. Pour them into your sprouting jar and fill the jar with water about ⅔ full, at least 1 inch above your sprouting agent of choice.
3. Allow to soak for 8-24 hours. Usually overnight is sufficient.
4. Drain, and allow to dry for about 8 hours.
5. Rinse and drain sprouts every 8-12 hours (about 2-3 times a day). After you drain, place your jar upside down at an angle (place it in a bowl to keep it properly propped).
6. Continue to rinse and drain as directed for 3-7 days or until sprouting has occurred. You may enjoy them with small or long sprouts. Each phase of the sprouting process may provide a different taste or bitterness so taste as you go and experiment!

A word about soaking

Soaking has similar benefits as sprouting. It is acceptable to simply soak your food overnight and then prepare in the morning, even without the presence of sprouts. I often do this, especially with my nuts.

MEAL IDEAS

<u>Grains</u>
(oats, wheat, buckwheat, rice, millet, barley, etc)

Low heat grains with nut milk and maple syrup for a healthy breakfast porridge.
Dry and grind grains down into a flour.
Cook grains on low heat in water and use as a base in meals such as stir-fries, curries,
buddha bowls and more.

<u>Nuts</u>
(almonds, cashews, walnuts, brazil nuts, etc)

Grind nuts into nut butters (see recipes)
Blend with water and strain for nut milks
Low heat in the oven with spices and enjoy as a snack

<u>Seeds</u>
(alfalfa, broccoli, radish, sunflower, quinoa etc)

Use sprouted seeds as a garnish on any salad, sandwich, wrap, soup, or enjoy alone. I
really enjoy the taste of alfalfa sprouts and broccoli sprouts.
Quinoa is great when low heated and used as a cereal porridge, a base for a veggie
dish, or sprinkled on a salad.

<u>Legumes / Beans</u>
(lentils, black beans, pinto beans, mung beans, chickpeas etc)

Add beans to any soup or chili.
Low heat beans and accompany with rice for a complete protein.
Sprinkle mung bean sprouts on a salad or sandwich.
Make sprouted hummus from chickpeas (see recipe)

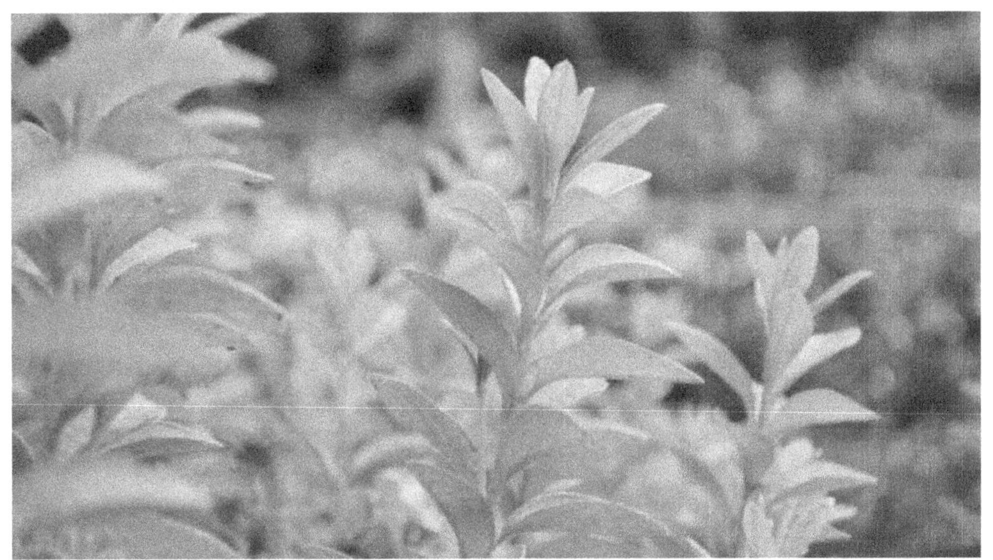

Fermentation

"In a world full of soda, be a kombucha"
-The internet, Pinterest probably

Bacteria is an often demonized living organism in the world today. Did you know that over 90% of the human body is comprised of bacteria? The world and environment we live in is full of beneficial bacteria that allow ecosystems to thrive, plants to grow, and life itself to exist. There is a misconception that bacteria is bad. Most bacteria is in fact very good, and necessary for you to stay alive. The key is in understanding how bacteria works, what it's role is, and how to nourish the presence of good bacteria while also avoiding the growth and contact with unproductive or harmful bacteria.

For the purposes of this ebook, we will focus now on the benefits of cultivating good bacteria in foods and how ingesting it is beneficial for the body. You are probably becoming familiar with the term "probiotics" and the trend it is becoming now to regularly ingest probiotic capsules. You may be pleased to learn that nature has its way of providing us with our very own naturally occurring probiotics - in food!

WHAT IS FERMENTING?

Fermenting is the process of cultivating or supporting the natural growth of beneficial microorganisms such as bacteria or yeast in foods. These organisms help to convert carbohydrates to alcohols or organic acids. Some examples of fermented foods are sauerkraut, pickles, miso, tempeh, kefir, yogurt, kombucha, sourdough, and kvass.

BENEFITS OF FERMENTATION

- High incidence of enzymes
- Presence of beneficial bacteria
- Natural preservation of foods

High incidence of enzymes

As noted in my chapter on Sprouting, enzymes are necessary for a healthful condition in the body. They are particularly helpful for the digestion of foods. Fermenting foods increases enzymes which will help to break down the food prior to ingestion, making it easier for the body to digest the food and absorb its nutrients.

Presence of beneficial bacteria

The ingestion of bacteria (especially from food sources) is helpful for improving gut health. Our gut is full of beneficial bacteria which is necessary for the breaking down and absorption of vitamins, minerals, fats, proteins and sugars. Bacteria also help to create certain nutrients for the body as well as serve as a line of defense against invaders such as pathogens and toxins found in the environment. Because of this, 75% of the immune system lives in the gut.

The high use of pharmaceuticals, antibiotics, exposure to toxins in the environment and poor eating habits such as the Standard American Diet (SAD) have all contributed to lower incidences of a healthy and diverse gut flora and higher incidences of poor gut health.. Because of this, many people are struggling with health problems linked to poor gut health such as (but not limited to): digestive problems, mental health problems, depression/anxiety, autoimmune disease, low-functioning immune system, chronic fatigue, chronic pain and inflammation, joint pain, skin conditions/rashes, acne, thyroid disorders, mood swings, insomnia, chronic fatigue, cancer, thyroid disease, hormone imbalance, infertility, PCOS, autoimmune disease and more. This is because the gut can become damaged and permeable, as well as lacking in its defenders (our friends, the bacteria) which leads to toxins, proteins and pathogens leaking out of the intestines and into the bloodstream. This condition of the bowels also causes poor nutrient absorption, therefore leading to deficiencies in the body. This can and does lead to systemic inflammation and chronic disease.

Not only is there a significant amount of science and anecdotal evidence to support this, but I personally have experienced the side effects of a damaged gut. My poor gut health was the first step in leading me down the path to autoimmune disease and overall chronic illness. One important step I took for healing my gut, and we can all take to healing our guts is introducing healthy bacteria to our bodies. Fermented foods are a great way to introduce a variety of wild strains of naturally occurring microorganisms that will nourish the gut, improve digestion, increase absorption, and ultimately improve health.

I prefer the use of fermented foods to probiotic supplements. Many supplements do not contain living or active bacteria, are limited to only 1-2 strains of bacteria (in comparison to hundreds available organically), are expensive, die upon reaching the acidic condition of the stomach and never reach the intestines, and can cause SIBO (small intestine bacterial overgrowth) by introducing an excess amount of isolated bacteria to the body. It's best to consult a naturopathic practitioner before using probiotic supplements.

Natural preservation of foods

During the fermentation process, the microorganisms create "bio-preservatives" such as alcohol, acetic acid and lactic acid which are able to preserve nutrients as well as prevent spoiling. They also prevent the growth of harmful bacteria by creating conditions that they cannot thrive in. Anciently, our predecessors used fermentation as a means of food preservation before there was access to refrigeration and other methods.

HOW TO FERMENT

The fermentation process varies widely between different foods. I am still in the early stages of learning how to ferment my own foods and anticipate I won't be a master by the time I want to complete this book. For that reason I'll provide a few simple recipes that I've experimented with and encourage you to do more personal research on all wonderful forms and methods for fermentation! I enjoy the Cultures for Health website, as well as the book "Fermentation for Dummies" by Marnie Wasserman.

In simple terms, almost all forms of fermentation begin by creating a brine (salt + water) that you allow your vegetables to sit in for an extended period of time (7 days - 7 months or longer!) An example of this kind of fermenting would be sauerkraut or pickles. Another method of fermentation is done by feeding a culture with a sugar and also allowing it to sit for an extended period of time. That sugar can be a lactose, fructose, sucrose or any other introduced or naturally occurring sugar, depending on what the "culture" of bacteria prefer. Examples of fermented foods using this method are kombucha, kefir and yogurt. Fermenting is as simple as giving bacteria or yeast favorable conditions to grow naturally. In my opinion is is like owning a cute little pet!

RECIPES

Sauerkraut

4 c green or red cabbage
1 tbsp sea salt

1. Wash and prepare cabbage. Cut into thin strips.
2. Sanitize bowl, utensils and mason jar that you'll be using to prepare the sauerkraut to prevent cross contamination.
3. Place cabbage in a bowl and sprinkle salt over it. Using hands, massage the cabbage leaves for several minutes until the salt draws out the water. Continue massaging until there is enough liquid to cover the cabbage leaves.
4. Spoon cabbage and its liquid into a pint sized mason jar. There should be enough liquid to cover the mixture at least ½ inch on top. Add a little bit of filtered water if necessary. It is important that all the cabbage leaves are completely submerged (to prevent mold).
5. Secure the lid of the mason jar and place in a room temperature or slightly cool and dark place (such as a cabinet or pantry).
6. Revisit the jar each day at least once a day and "burp" the lid. Burping the lid means slightly twisting it and releasing the gasses that have built up in the jar. Neglecting to do this can cause the jar to break.
7. Repeat the burping process daily and allow to sit for at least 7 days. At this point, taste your cabbage and see how you like it. The longer you allow it to sit, the more "fermented" it will taste. When it has reached the taste you like, put it in the fridge.

Options:

You can add any veggies to this mixture. I have enjoyed adding grated carrots, jalapenos, grated zucchini, or mixing red and green cabbage. The world is your oyster.

<u>Meal ideas:</u>

Serve on top of a salad, enjoy on a piece of avocado toast, with organic eggs, stir into cooled miso soup, piece onto pulp crackers, mix into any dip or dressing, eat it with a fork! Drink the juice for a health gut tonic and to help and upset or acidic stomach.

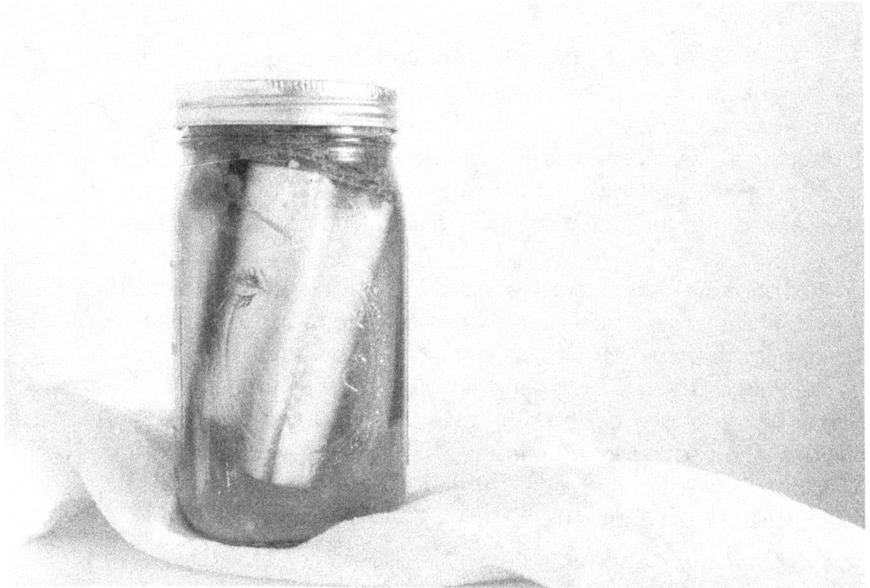

Dill Pickles

1-2 cucumbers
¼ c fresh dill
3 bay leaves
3 cloves garlic
1 heaping tbsp sea salt
½ tsp black pepper
16 oz filtered water

Optional:
Mustard seeds, peppercorns, red pepper flakes

Sanitize a pint sized mason jar and any other materials you use to prevent cross contamination.

1. First, you will want to make the brine. Stir your heaping tablespoon of salt into the water and stir. Set aside and allow to dissolve.
2. Wash, prepare and cut your cucumbers into long strips. Layer your mason jar with dill, bay leaves, crushed garlic, and pepper. Add all other ingredients you choose to as well. Stuff in your cucumbers lengthwise over them until they are tightly packed into the jar. You want it to be difficult for them to float to the top.
3. Pour your brine over the cucumbers and fill until it is about ½ inch from the top. If you find that your cucumbers keep floating to the top, use a couple bay leaves and lay them over top to keep the cucumbers submerged.
4. Screw your lid on the mason jar and set in a room temperature dark place. Each day, visit your pickles and slightly unscrew the lid to "burp" it and release the gasses. Allow to ferment for around 1 week. Taste your pickles at this point and allow to ferment for longer for more flavor. When you have reached your desired taste, place it in the fridge.

<u>Meal ideas:</u>

Eat alone, enjoy on the side of a black bean burger and homemade fries, slice and enjoy in a salad, drink the juice as a healthy gut tonic.

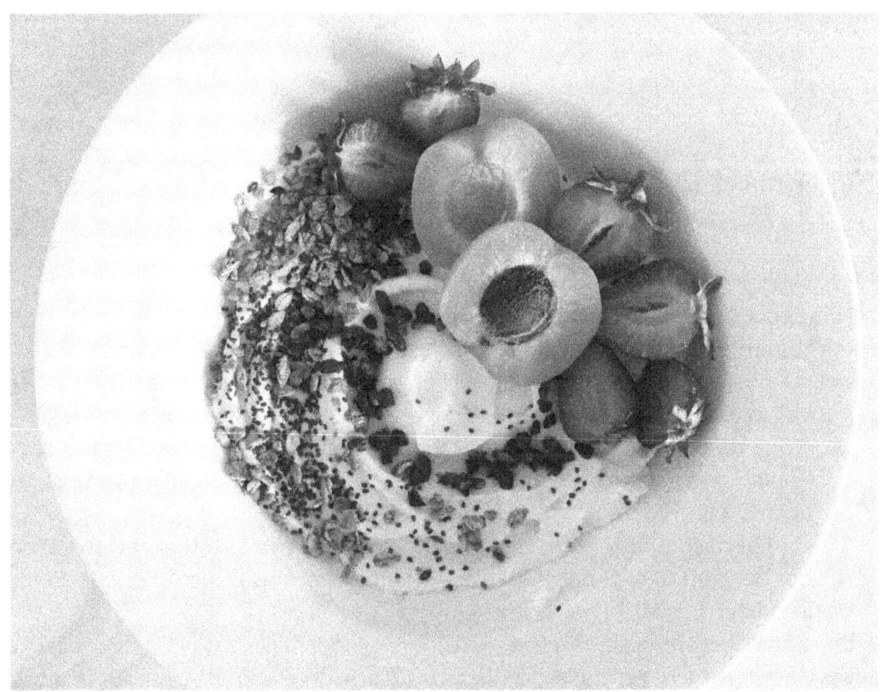

Coconut Yogurt

2 c of homemade coconut milk (or 1 can full fat, unsweetened coconut milk)
1 tsp probiotic powder (2-3 capsules)

Optional:
Raw honey or maple syrup to sweeten after fermentation.
3 tbsp arrowroot flour/starch

1. Sanitize the materials you'll be using to make the yogurt to prevent cross contamination.
2. Pour coconut milk into a glass mason jar. Add probiotic powder and mix until combined! Cover top with a piece of paper towel or natural cotton and secure with a rubber band.
3. Allow to sit in a room temperature place for at least 8 hours. A good place to put it is in the oven (with it off), with the light on. This will help to maintain a good temperature.
4. The longer it sits, the more fermented it will taste! Check the mixture at 8 hours and refrigerate if it is to your liking, or allow to sit longer for more flavor.

Stir in sweetener if desired. This method will yield a very "runny" yogurt, which would work best in smoothies or for drinking.

<u>For thicker yogurt:</u>
1. Heat coconut milk in a pan over medium heat. Whisk in arrowroot flour until combined and lower heat to a simmer until mixture thickens. It will yield a gooey texture but don't worry, it will change during fermentation.
2. Allow mixture to cool to room temperature. In a separate bowl, whisk probiotic powder with a little water until combined. Add probiotics to coconut and whisk. It is important that the coconut mixture isn't too hot or the probiotics will die!
3. Store in a mason jar at room temperature with a paper towel or natural cotton rubber banded over the lid. Follow same instructions as listed above to reach desired flavor.
4. Once it's done fermenting the mixture may look a little clumpy. Empty into a bowl and use a hand mixer to blend until smooth, about 1-2 minutes (you could also use a blender). Add in sweetener if desired and mix again! Enjoy.

<u>Yogurt starter!</u>
Before adding sweetener or serving, remove ¼ c of the yogurt and save it in the fridge as a "starter" for your next batch. To make more yogurt, simply remove starter several hours before and allow to come to room temperature and then stir into your coconut milk in place of probiotics. Follow the above steps.

<u>Meal ideas:</u>
Serve with homemade granola and sliced fruit on top with a drizzle of raw honey, blend into smoothies, if you didn't add sweetener - use as a vegan "sour cream", use in place of greek yogurt for any recipe, pour into smoothies for a creamy probiotic boost!

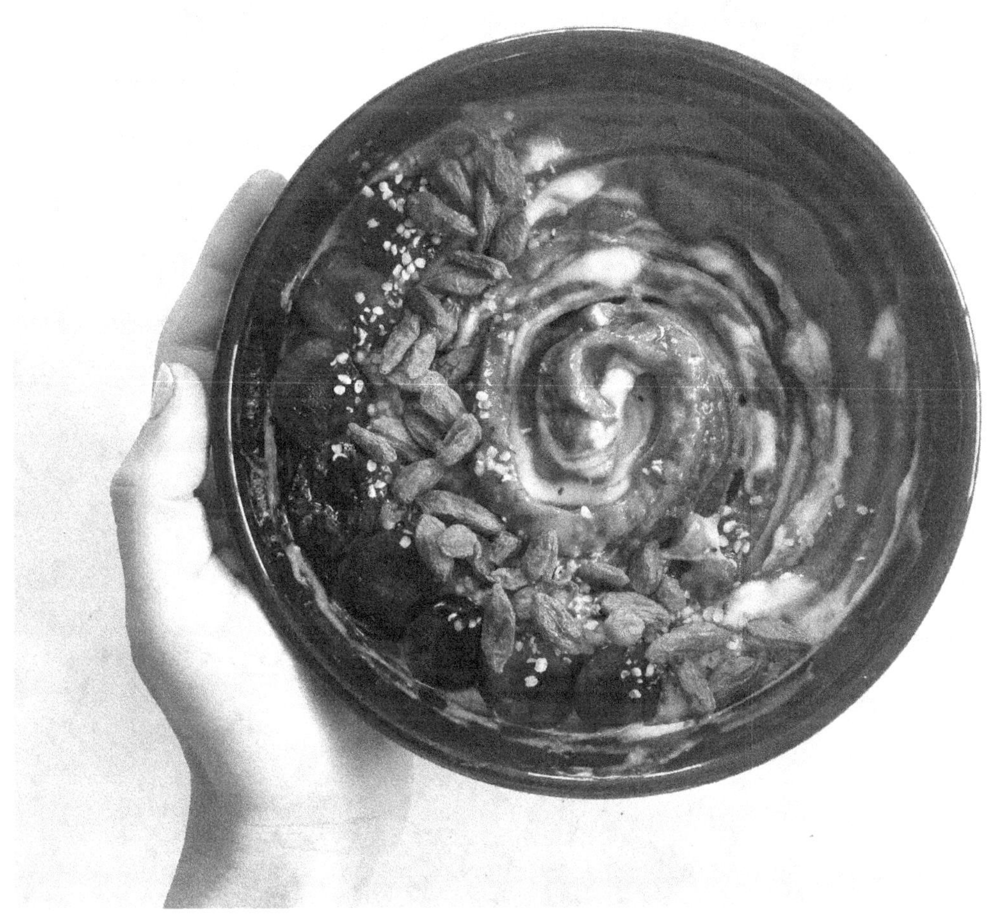

Recipes

"Eat like you love yourself"
-Unknown

This book originally started out as a recipe book and morphed into so much more! I wanted a place to share some of my absolutely favorite recipes I have made over the years while I have healed my body using whole foods. I know how difficult it can be to start transitioning to a healthy lifestyle and to know what to eat or where to start. Most of the foods I enjoy are very simple and plain. I honestly love fruits and vegetables by themselves. But along the way I found myself craving a lot of comfort foods and that was the most difficult part! Because of that, I created a lot of replacements for my favorite unhealthy foods so that I could still feel like I was indulging and enjoying a rich life while also avoiding the inflammatory effects. I have been able to maintain a lifestyle of healthy intuitive eating because I try to enjoy what I eat and not restrict myself. I wanted to share the very recipes that have become my comfort foods and helped me truly enjoy eating healthy.

Because of that, not all of these recipes are going to use perfect methods of nutrient preservation. Many of them do, but others of them simply serve as a healthy alternative to some of my favorite treats or savory dishes. I also have shaped most of my recipes around my own personal intuitive eating, moral values and preferences. Because of that, these recipes do not call for any animal products like meat or dairy and most of them are also gluten-free. There are lots of meat based recipe books and pinterest so I feel that the best thing I can share is how to utilize and enjoy more plant foods. I try to provide different options that you can try substituting to honor your own intuitive eating as well. Feel free to add or take away ingredients. Use your best judgement to decide how to adapt the recipes to what makes you happy!

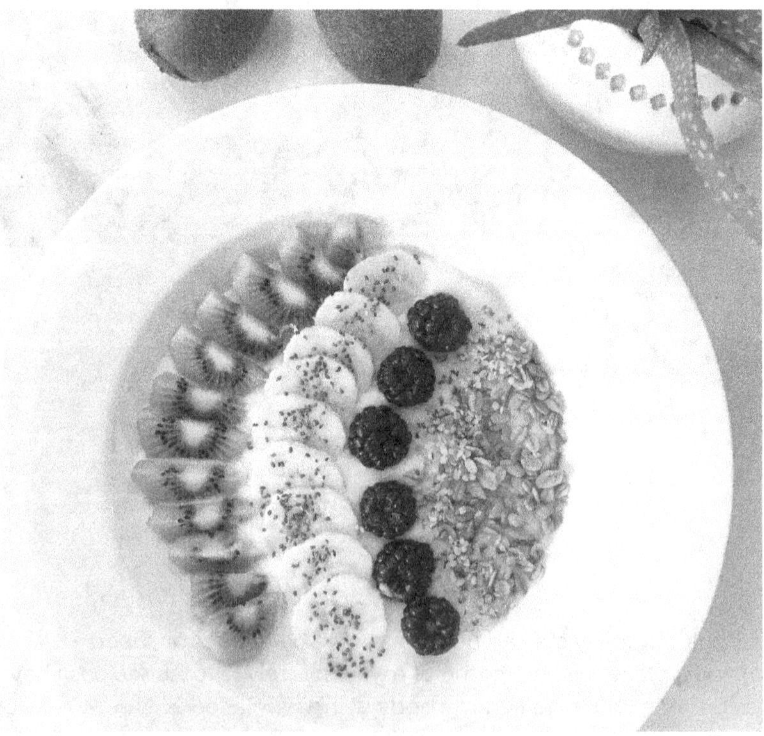

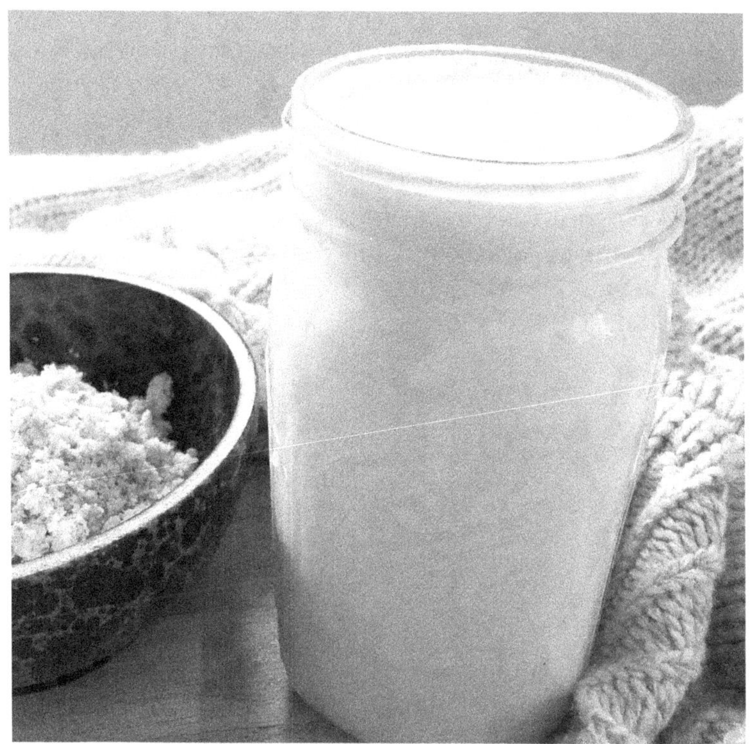

Almond Milk

2 c raw almonds
6-8 c filtered water
1 tsp vanilla extract
Dash sea salt

1. Soak almonds overnight 8-12 hours.
2. Drain and rinse almonds, and then slide skins off setting the blanched almond aside.
3. Add blanched almonds to blender and add all ingredients. Blend on high for 1-3 minutes until combined. Pour mixture through a nut bag into a glass container and strain the pulp and squeeze all the liquid out.. Almond milk will last in fridge for 3-4 days.

Meal ideas:

Use as liquid base in smoothies, over fresh granola (see recipe), in baking, as a replacement for anything that calls for dairy milk, as a refreshing beverage

Almond milk should become the best friend to anyone who loves milk but desires to upgrade to a healthier alternative. Almonds provide a slightly sweet, but nutty-undertone to the milk that goes undetected in cooking and baking while also providing the same results. This nut is one of the most nutrient dense in the nut family as it is rich in minerals.

Cacao Almond Milk

2 c raw almonds
6-8 c filtered water
6 tbsp cacao powder
1 tbsp raw honey
1 tbsp coconut oil
1 tsp vanilla extract
Dash sea salt

1. Soak almonds overnight 8-12 hours.
2. Drain and rinse almonds, and then slide skins off setting the blanched almond aside.
3. Add blanched almonds to blender with water. Blend on high for 1-3 minutes until combined. Pour mixture through a nut bag into a glass container, strain the pulp and squeeze until liquid is out.
4. Return the liquid to the blender and add remaining ingredients. Blend on high for an additional 1 minute or until combined. Return to glass container. Almond milk will last in fridge for 3-4 days.

Meal ideas:

Use as liquid base for warm elixirs (see recipes), use as base in smoothies, as a healthy alternative to chocolate milk, blended with frozen bananas for nice cream

Hemp Milk

3-4 tbsp hemp seeds
6-8 c filtered water
1 tsp vanilla extract
Dash sea salt

1. Blend all ingredients in high speed blender for 1-3 minutes or until combined. Strain through a nut milk bag into a glass container. Enjoy for 3-4 days in the fridge.

Meal ideas:

As a base for smoothies, as a nutritious milk for toddlers who have weaned from breastmilk, in overnight oats (see recipe)

Hemp seeds are an excellent source of plant protein. They are a complete protein, meaning that they contain all 9 essential amino acids! They also possess omega-3 and omega-6 fatty acids, which are essential to get through food as they are not made in the body. The omega-3 fatty acids are especially good for brain health. Consume hemp seeds if you struggle with mental illness or hormone imbalance for nourishment. This food is also an excellent anti-inflammatory! Just as it's fully developed plant, Cannabis, hemp seeds also have a wide range of medicinal benefits.

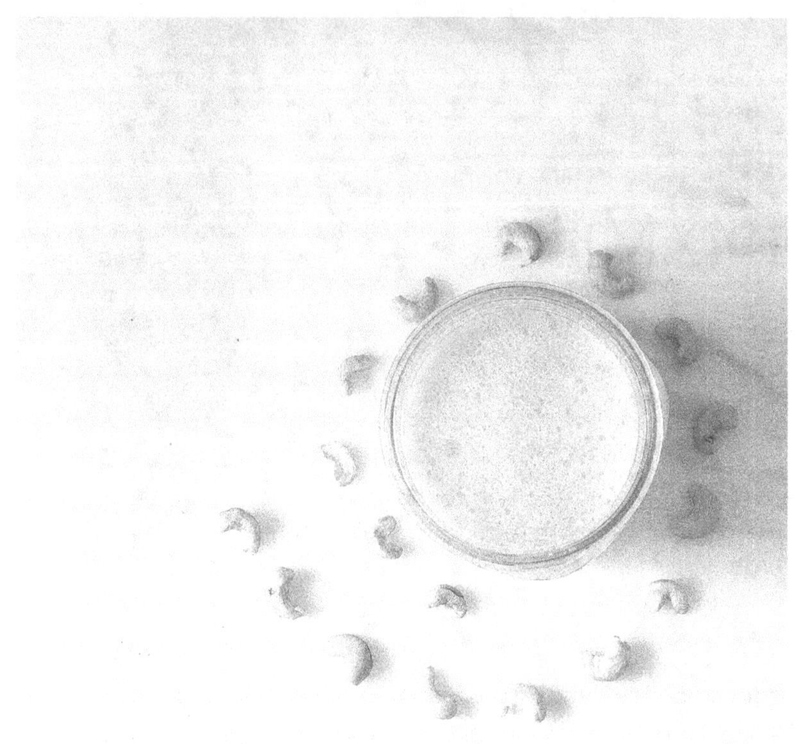

Sweet Cashew Milk

3 c raw cashews
6-8 c filtered water
1 tsp vanilla extract
1 tbsp raw honey or maple syrup
Dash sea salt

1. Soak cashews overnight or at least 3 hours.
2. Drain and rinse cashews. Add cashews to blender and add all ingredients except sweetener. Blend on high for 1-3 minutes until combined. Pour mixture through a nut bag into a glass container, strain the pulp and squeeze until liquid is out.

3. Pour liquid back into the blender and add honey. Blend on high for an
    additional 1 minute, and then return to glass container. Cashew milk will last
    in fridge for 3-4 days.

<u>Meal ideas:</u>
As a base for teas and elixirs (see recipes), in homemade nice cream, top with
cinnamon and enjoy alone, on the side to wash down muffins (see recipes)

Flax Milk

3-4 tbsp flax seeds
6-8 c filtered water
1 tsp vanilla extract
Dash sea salt

1. Blend all ingredients on high for 1-3 minutes or until combined. Strain
    through a nut milk bag into a glass container. Enjoy for 3-4 days in the fridge.

<u>Meal ideas:</u>

As a base for overnight oats (see recipe), in baking, as a healthy milk alternative for a
toddler who has weaned from breastmilk, in smoothies (see recipes!)

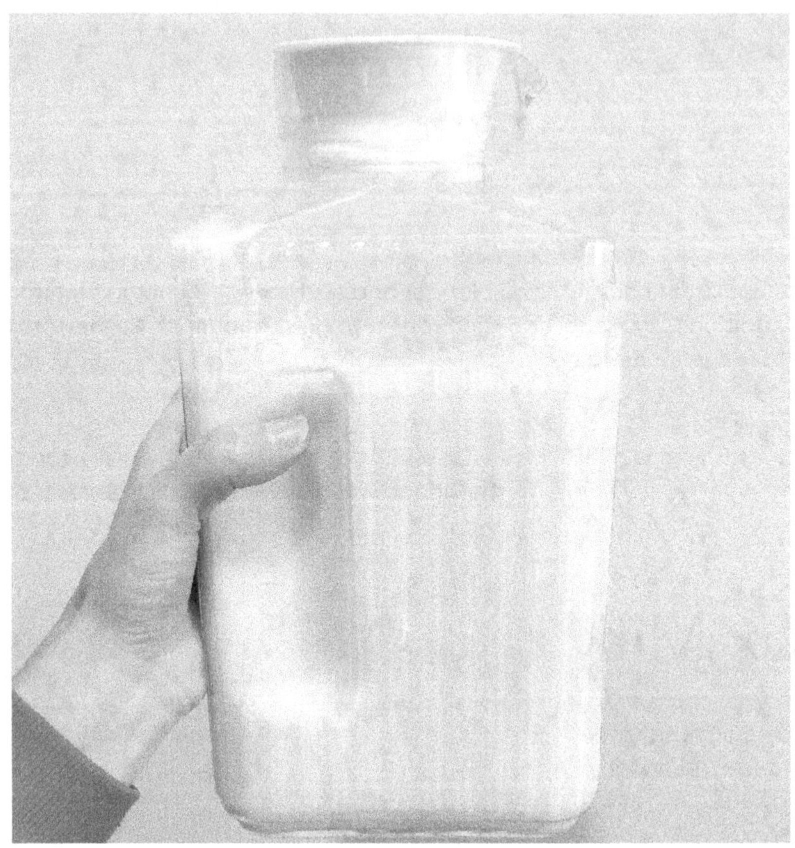

Sweet Oat Milk

2 c organic rolled oats
8 c purified water
1-2 tbsp maple syrup
1 tsp vanilla extract
Dash sea salt

1. Blend all ingredients except sweetner on high for 1-3 minutes or until combined. Strain through a nut milk bag into a glass container. Return to blender and add maple syrup, blend for 30 more seconds and return to glass container.

<u>Meal Ideas:</u>

Warm up with cinnamon and enjoy alone, as a base in smoothies or elixirs (see recipes!)

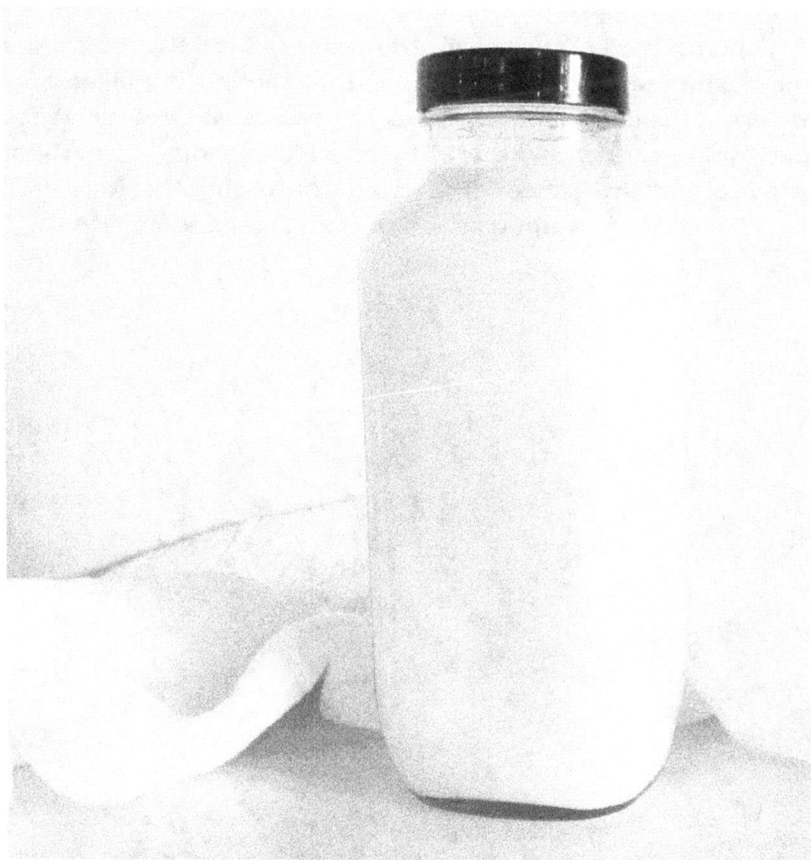

Coconut Milk

2 c unsweetened shredded coconut
6-8 c purified water

1. Blend all ingredients on high for 1-3 minutes or until combined. Strain through a nut milk bag into a glass container. Enjoy for 3-4 days in the fridge.

<u>Meal ideas:</u>

Freeze for homemade nicecream (see recipe), in curries and soups, as a healthy alternative to milk for toddlers who have weaned from breastmilk, as a base for smoothies

Coconut is an extremely nutrient dense food that often goes underestimated. High vitamin C and B vitamins as well as essential minerals, the coconut also serves as natures electrolyte (especially when drinking coconut water). The humble coconut has anti-bacterial, anti-viral and anti-cancer properties. Consuming this food regularly will also nourish healthy skin, hair and nails.

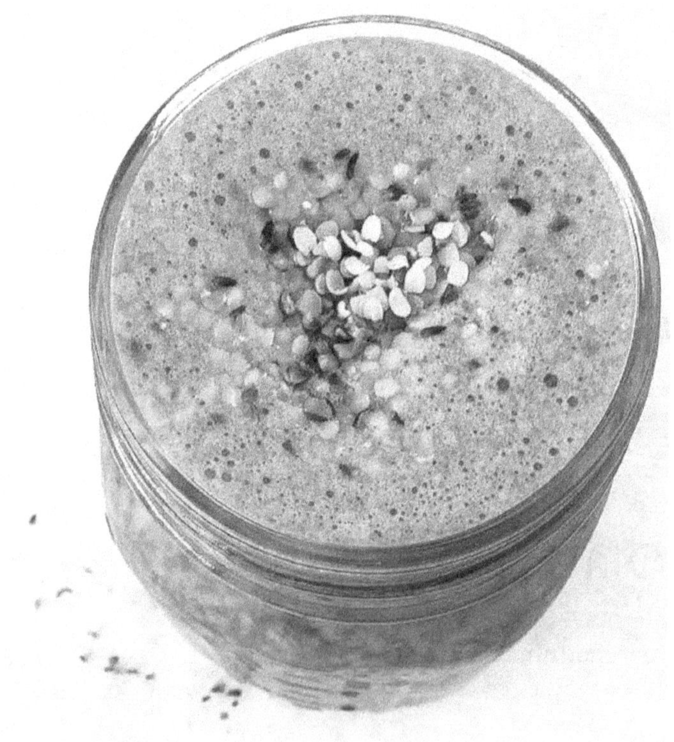

SMOOTHIES

One of my all-time favorite healthy hacks is adding vegetables to my smoothies. Especially for picky toddlers and spouses! Some of my favorites to have on hand are:

Sweet Potatoes
Zucchini
Cauliflower
Broccoli
Butternut squash
Leafy greens

You'll want to prepare them by first, by cutting them into 1-2" chunks. Then steaming them (except the greens). Use a steam basket in a pot of simmering water and leave veggies in the basket with the lid on for about 15-20 minutes or until soft. Lay the veggies out on a baking sheet covered in parchment paper and freeze for 2-3 hours. Remove from baking sheet and put into a plastic bag or container. This method prevents them from sticking together!

Any veggie can be added to a smoothie, but keep in mind it will change the texture. Add banana or a scoop of nut butter to help mitigate the texture and dates to help sweeten if necessary.

The first healthy foods I introduced into my diet were smoothies. Even in my darkest days, I've always been able to stomach a nourishing and energy-boosting smoothie. They can be adapted to meet the needs of almost any taste buds, from a picky toddler to a sensitive tummy. If you're feeling overwhelmed about healthy eating and want to know where to start, try making one smoothie a day and I promise you'll feel the difference!

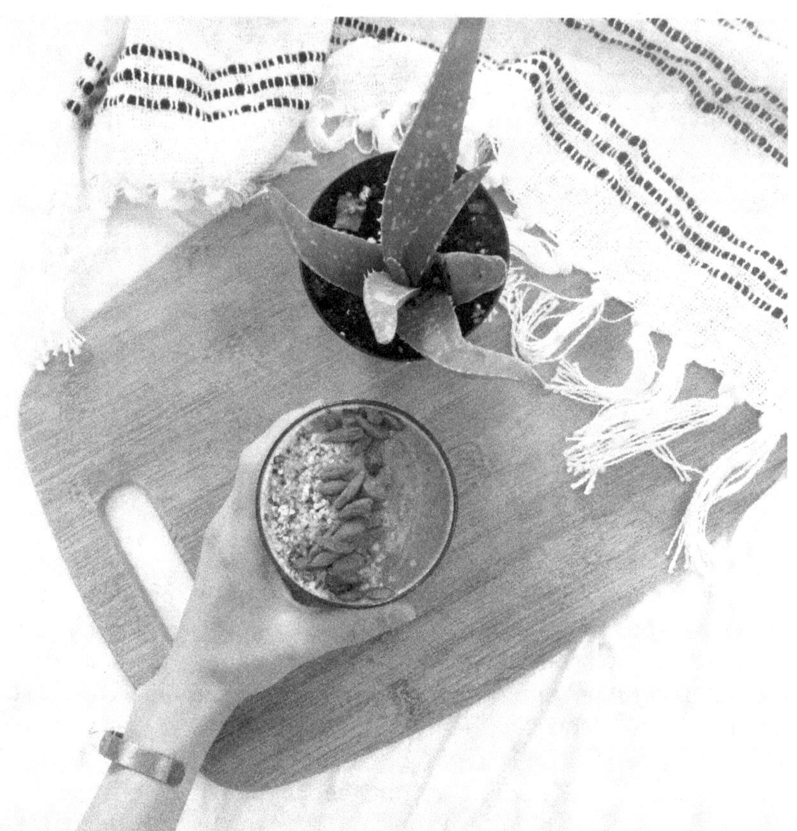

Hemp Green Smoothie

2-3 bananas (frozen optional)
4 dates
3 tbsp hemp seeds
1-2 c spinach leaves
1-2 c nut milk
Handful ice cubes
Dash ceylon cinnamon

Add all ingredients to a high speed blender and blend on high for 1-2 minutes until combined. If you don't have a high speed blender, soak dates for 20 minutes prior to blending your smoothie. Ice cubes not necessary if your bananas are frozen.

Serve in a glass jar for breakfast or as a treat.
This smoothie can be used as a "base" for any smoothie. It's full proof. Add fruits and veggies and it will still taste delicious! Experiment to find what tastes you enjoy.

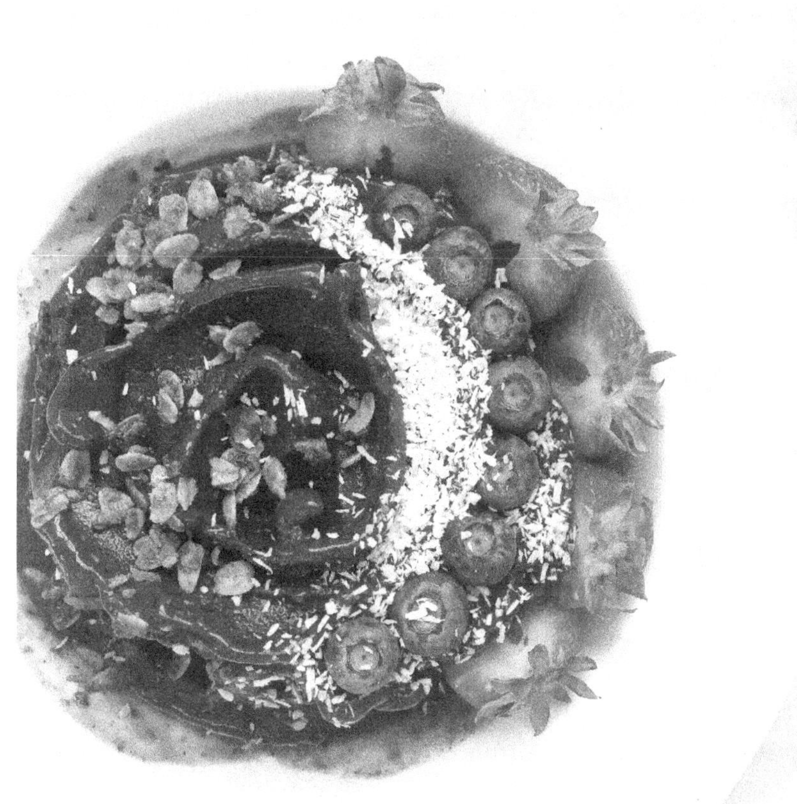

Antioxidant Smoothie

1-2 bananas
1.5 c frozen mixed berries
        (strawberries, blueberries, blackberries, raspberries)
½ c baby kale
1 tbsp hemp seeds
1 tbsp chia seeds

1/2 tsp hawaiian spirulina
1-2 c nut mlk

Add all ingredients in a high speed blender and blend for 1-3 minutes or until completely combined. Enjoy in a glass or bowl with granola sprinkled on top.

Berries are among the most antioxidant rich foods in the plant kingdom. Antioxidants help to restore cell damage, fight free radicals, and reduce inflammation. Berries help us to heal on a cellular level. They are also very delicious and if you struggle to eat fresh produce before it goes bad - berries are even better frozen!

Tropical Breeze

1-2 bananas
1.5 c frozen tropical fruit
        (pineapple, mango, and papaya)
½ grapefruit, squeezed juice
½ c orange juice
½-1 c nut milk milk

Add all ingredients in a high speed blender and blend for 1-3 minutes or until completely combined.

Choco Cherry Smoothie

1-2 bananas
1 c frozen cherries
1 c spinach leaves
1-2 tbsp cacao powder
2 dates
1-2 c nut milk
1 tbsp hemp seeds

Add all ingredients in a high speed blender and blend for 1-3 minutes or until completely combined. If you don't have a high speed blender, allow dates to soak for 20 minutes prior to blending.

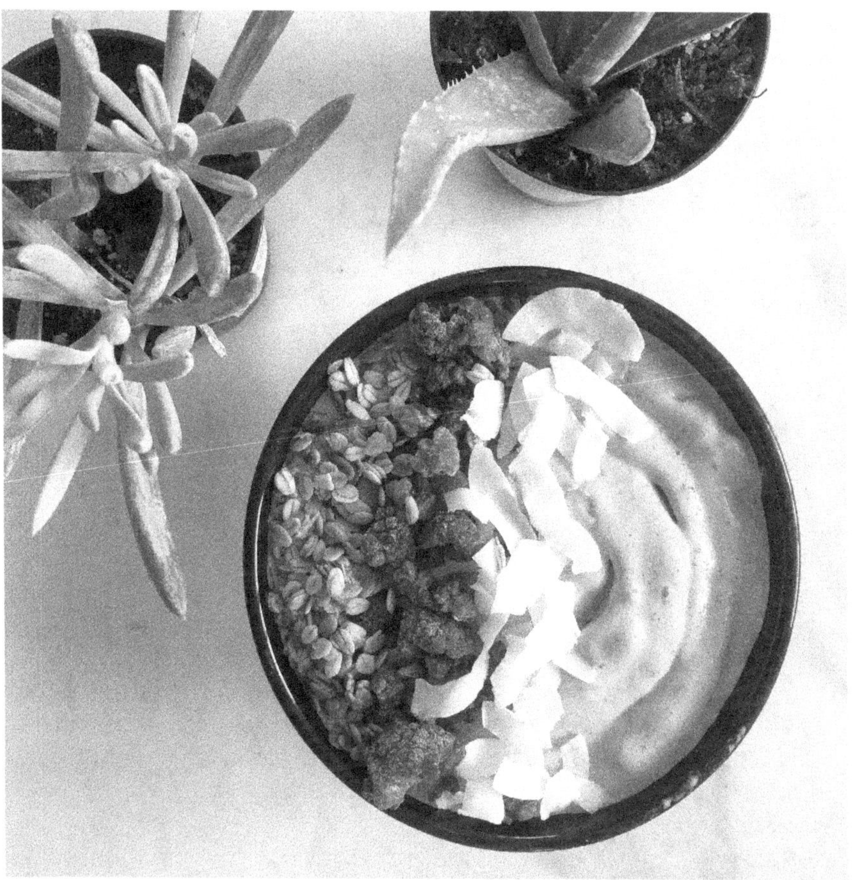

Sweet Potato Smoothie

1-2 bananas
½ c frozen raspberries
½ c frozen strawberries
½-1 c steamed and frozen sweet potato
1 tbsp hemp seeds
1 tbsp flax seeds
1-2 c nut milk

1. To prepare sweet potato for the smoothie, steam or bake sweet potato until soft. Spread onto a baking sheet covered in parchment paper and freeze. Then add to a plastic bag or container to hold in the freezer until ready!
2. Add all ingredients in a high speed blender and blend for 1-3 minutes or until completely combined. Enjoy with fresh fruit and granola on top.

Veggie Smoothie

1 banana (optional)
1 c frozen blueberries
1 c steamed and frozen cauliflower
¼ c steamed and frozen sweet potato
1 inch zucchini
½ c baby kale
1 tbsp almond butter
1 tbsp flax seeds
Dash ceylon cinnamon
1-2 c almond milk

1. To prepare cauliflower and sweet potato for the smoothie, steam or bake them until soft. Spread onto a baking sheet covered in parchment paper and freeze. Then add to a plastic bag or container to hold in the freezer until ready!
2. Add all ingredients in a high speed blender and blend for 1-3 minutes or until completely combined. Smoothie is subtly sweet so add sweetener if necessary.

I created the "veggie smoothie" (creative name right?) when I was struggling with intense inflammation. It was during this time that even fruit sugars would upset my stomach. I have always felt that smoothies are the easiest way to get in a lot of fruits and vegetables when it's harder to eat them otherwise, especially if you don't have the taste for them. This smoothie was a life saver because it is lower in fruit sugars and still tastes good if you leave out the banana! I ate this smoothie almost every day when I couldn't eat anything else. I hold a special place in my heart for the veggie smoothie, so I hope it finds someone who is feeling down

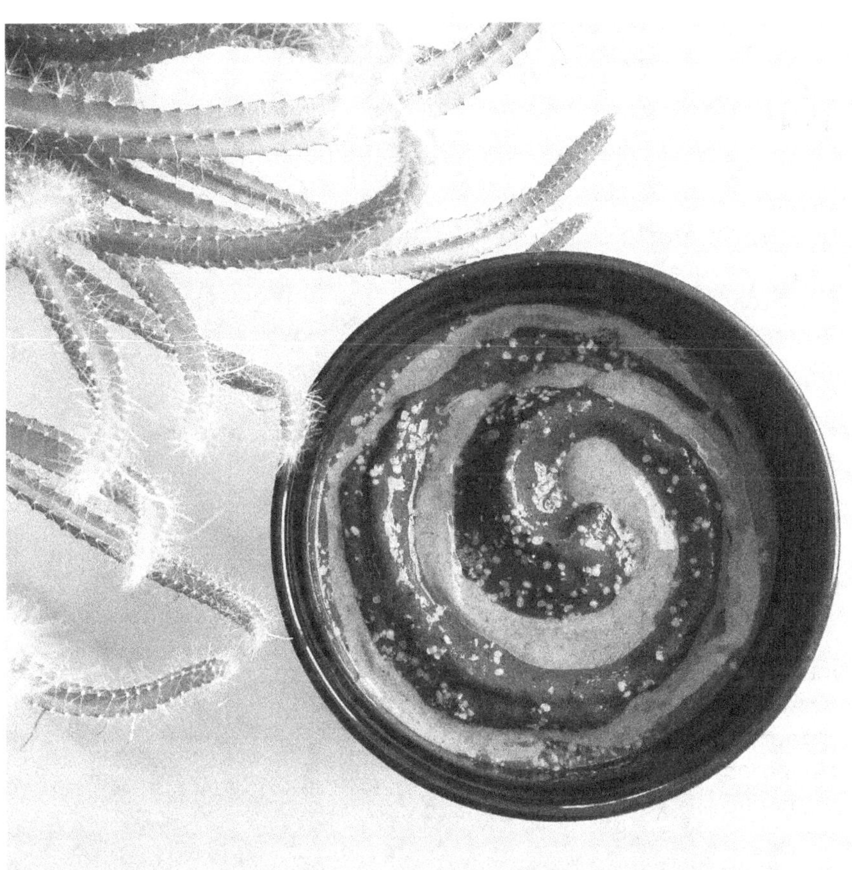

PB&J Smoothie

1 banana
1.5 c berries (strawberries or raspberries are yum!)
2 tbsp natural peanut butter
1 tbsp flax seeds
1 tbsp chia seeds
1 c nut milk

Add all ingredients in a high speed blender and blend for 1-3 minutes or until completely combined.

Choco-Peanut Butter Protein Shake

2 frozen bananas
1-2 tbsp peanut butter
1 tbsp cacao powder
1 scoop chocolate plant based protein powder
1 handful spinach
¼ c rolled oats

Add all ingredients in a high speed blender and blend for 1-3 minutes or until completely combined.

Mango Lassi

1 banana
1.5 c frozen mango
½ c coconut yogurt
Dash cinnamon
Dash turmeric
Dash ginger
½ c nut milk

Add all ingredients in a high speed blender and blend for 1-3 minutes or until completely combined. Serve on the side of an Indian curry for a fun and cultural dish.

Carrot Apple Ginger Juice

6 large carrots
1 apple (any variety)

1 inch ginger root

Push all ingredients through a juicer. If you don't have one, add all ingredients to a high speed blender with about 2-3 c of filtered water and strain through a nut milk bag. Makes 1 glass.

Juicing is a great way to eat foods in their raw, living form. I love drinking juices especially when I am feeling ill or when I have noticed I haven't eaten enough produce during the day. If you struggle to keep produce from going bad, consider juicing them when they are on their last day to quickly use them up without waste! Make sure that if you drink fruit/vegetable juices that you always chew and swish each sip! This helps to initiate digestion by firing up the salivary glands and digestive juices in your stomach. You will digest and absorb the nutrients of the juice better this way and it will reduce the spike in blood sugar.

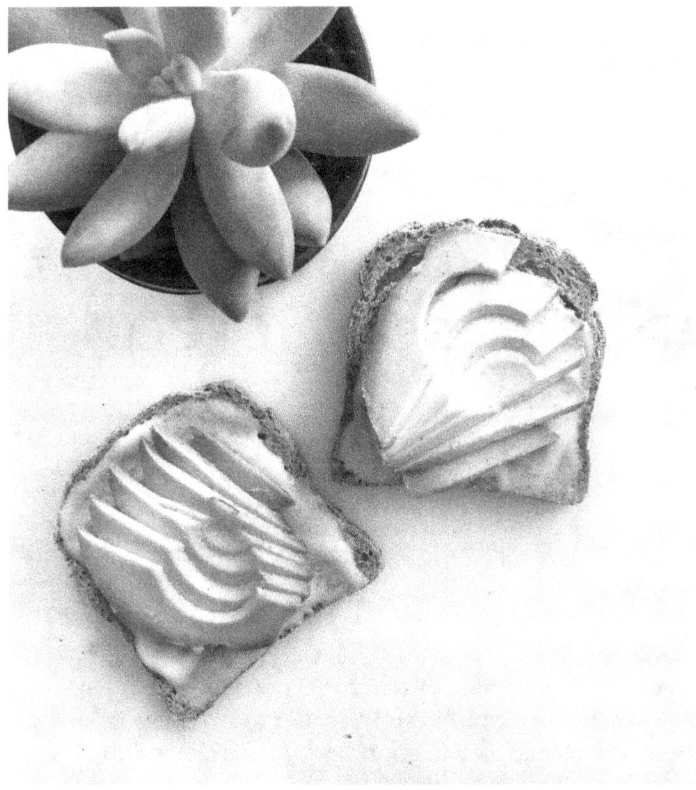

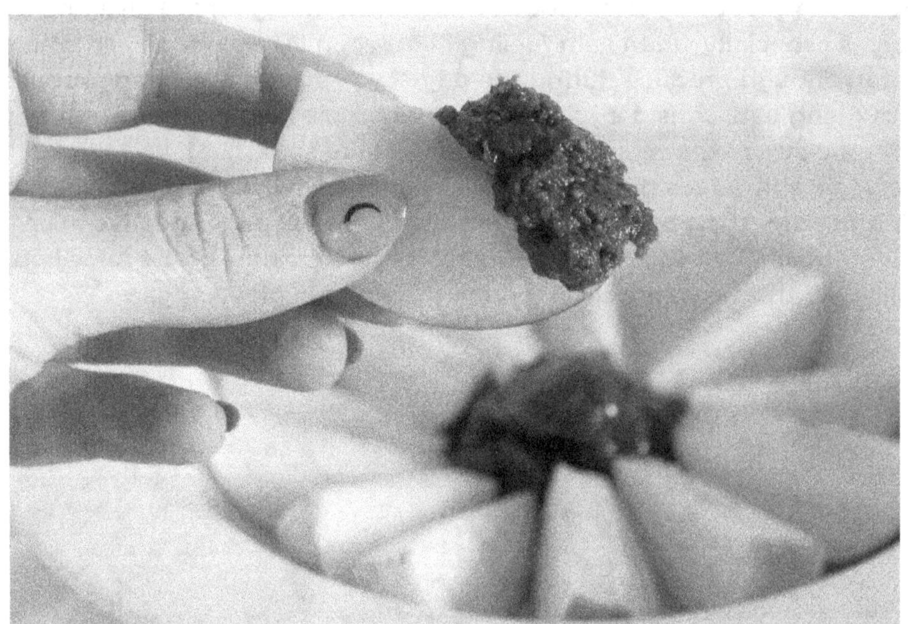

Hazelnut Cacao Spread
(almost-nutella)

3 c roasted hazelnuts
3 tbsp cacao powder
2 tbsp coconut oil or olive oil*
1 tbsp maple syrup
½ tsp sea salt

1. Preheat oven to 350 degrees F. Roast for 15 mins.
2. Once nuts have cooled, rub skins off and add to a high speed blender with oil until smooth. Add cacao and salt and slowly add maple syrup to desired taste/consistency. Store in fridge.

*coconut oil will reap a harder consistency when refrigerated. Olive oil will be softer. Use whatever oil will provide your preferred consistency, or leave out of fridge for best results.

<u>Snack ideas:</u>

With sliced apples, as a fruit dip, on a piece of toast, spread over muffins, on top of nice cream, or eat plain with a spoon!

Honey Roasted Peanut butter

3 c roasted peanuts
1.5 tbsp coconut oil or olive oil*
1 tbsp raw honey

Add peanuts to a high speed blender with oil and blend until smooth. Add honey and blend again until combined. Store in fridge.

*coconut oil will reap a harder consistency when refrigerated. Olive oil will be softer. Use whatever oil will provide your preferred consistency, or leave out of fridge for best results.

<u>Snack Ideas:</u>

With sliced apples, spread over crackers, in peanut thai sauce (see recipe), in seed power bites (see recipe), in smoothies, over toast with sliced banana and cinnamon, with a spoon!

Raw (unpasteurized, unfiltered) honey is truly the nectar of life. It contains living probiotics and enzymes that help to build and strengthen the gut flora. Raw honey is known to help treat seasonal allergies! It is also anti-bacterial and will help to soothe an upset stomach. Raw honey is my favorite sweetener!

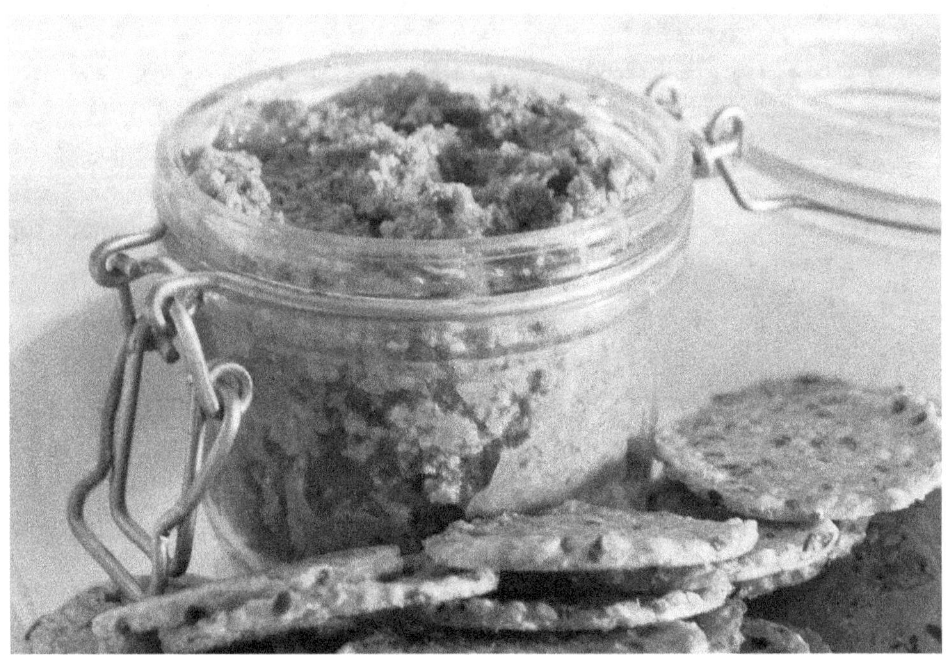

Almond Butter

3 c raw almonds
1 tbsp coconut or olive oil*
½ tsp sea salt (optional)

Roast almonds on a baking sheet lined with parchment paper at 350 degrees F for 15 mins. Let cool, add to blender with oil and salt and blend until smooth.

*coconut oil will reap a harder consistency when refrigerated. Olive oil will be softer. Use whatever oil will provide your preferred consistency, or leave out of fridge for best results.

<u>Snack Ideas:</u>

Fruit dip for bananas, apples or berries, in smoothies, spread over toast with hemp seeds, to make granola (see granola recipe), and… with a spoon of course.

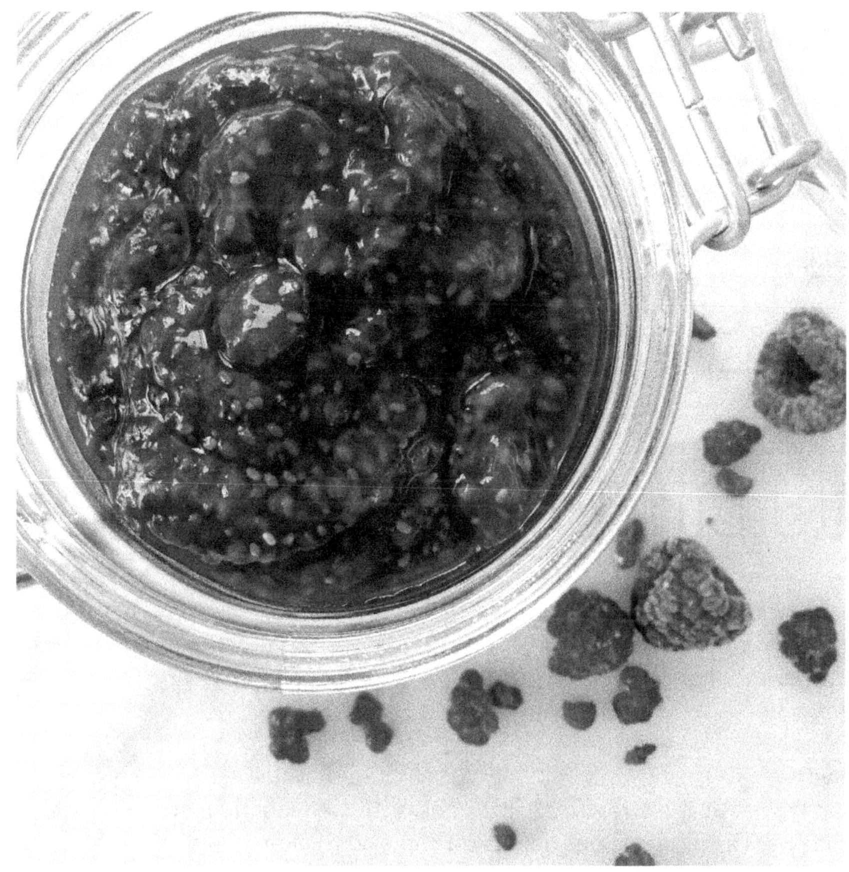

Raspberry Chia Jam

2 c frozen organic raspberries
1 tbsp fresh squeezed lemon juice
1 tbsp chia seeds
1 tbsp raw honey or maple syrup

1. Place a small pot over medium heat. Add raspberries, lemon juice, and sweetner. Stir until mixture begins to bubble. Reduce to low heat & allow to simmer for 10 minutes, stirring occasionally. Raise heat back to medium, until mixture begins to bubble again. Allow to bubble for 3-5 minutes, until mixture seems to begin to thicken.

2. Remove from heat & stir in chia seeds.
3. Allow mixture to cool before pouring into a glass container. Keep in fridge.

<u>Snack ideas:</u>

Spread over toast or rice cake, dollop over coconut yogurt and granola, drizzle over homemade nice cream

Wild Blueberry Syrup

1 c frozen wild blueberries
2 tbsp pure maple syrup
1 tbsp arrowroot flour/starch
Filtered water

Options:
You can leave out the arrowroot, all it does is thicken it a bit. I often make it without out of laziness and it's still delicious. You can also thicken it with chia seeds (1-2 tbsp).

1. Place frozen blueberries into a small saucepan and warm over medium heat. Continue simmering until berries dethaw into a watery mixture.
2. Add arrowroot to a little water and whisk together. Stir into blueberry mixture.
3. Add maple syrup, and continue whisking until combined.
4. Lower heat to low simmer and add more liquid for desired consistency.

<u>Meal ideas:</u>

Pour over buckwheat waffles (see recipe), drizzle over nicecream, use as a jam spread on toast

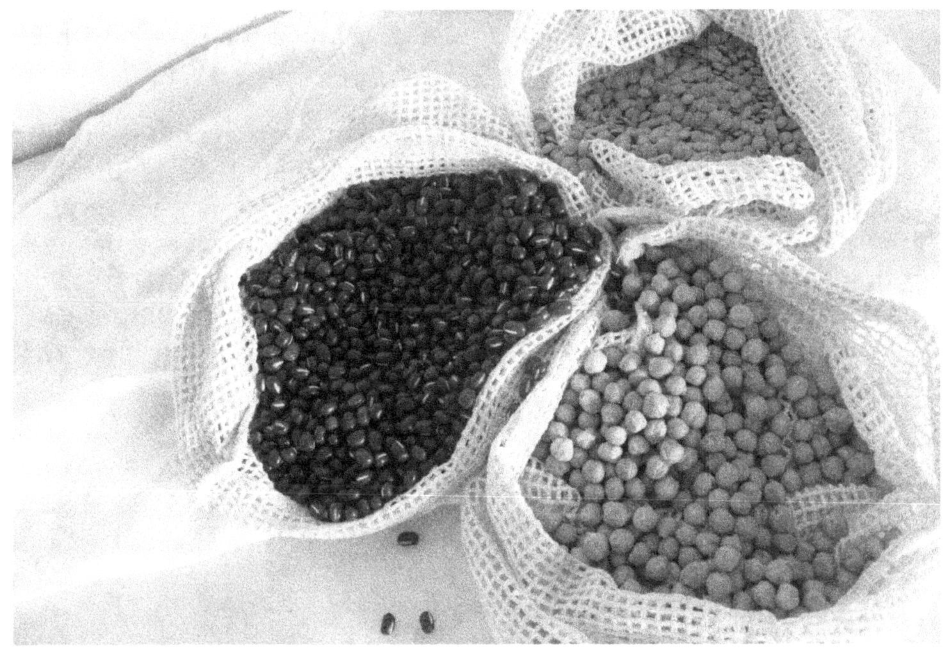

Sprouted Hummus

1.5 c organic sprouted chick peas (or 1 can chickpeas)
1 tbsp lemon juice
1-2 cloves of garlic
2 tbsp tahini *optional*
½ tsp cumin
½ tsp salt
½ tsp pepper
Filtered water
Olive oil
Paprika

1. Place all ingredients in a blender or food processor except olive oil and paprika. Blend on high until combined.
2. Add more or less spices to taste, and water for desired consistency.
3. Serve with drizzle of olive oil and dash of paprika.

<u>Snack ideas:</u>

Serve with raw veggies, eat with avocado toast, spread on a wrap or sandwich, blend into a veggie soup, enjoy with pulp crackers (see recipe)

As I mentioned earlier in the book - chickpeas was one of the mystery foods that had me running to the bathroom within 20 minutes! A hummus girl at heart I was disappointed to make this discovery. As discussed in my chapter on sprouting, the sprouting process makes it so that I am able to easily digest the hummus! It is one of my favorite "snack" foods as it can make almost anything appeal to the salty and savory cravings I have while also providing some nourishment.

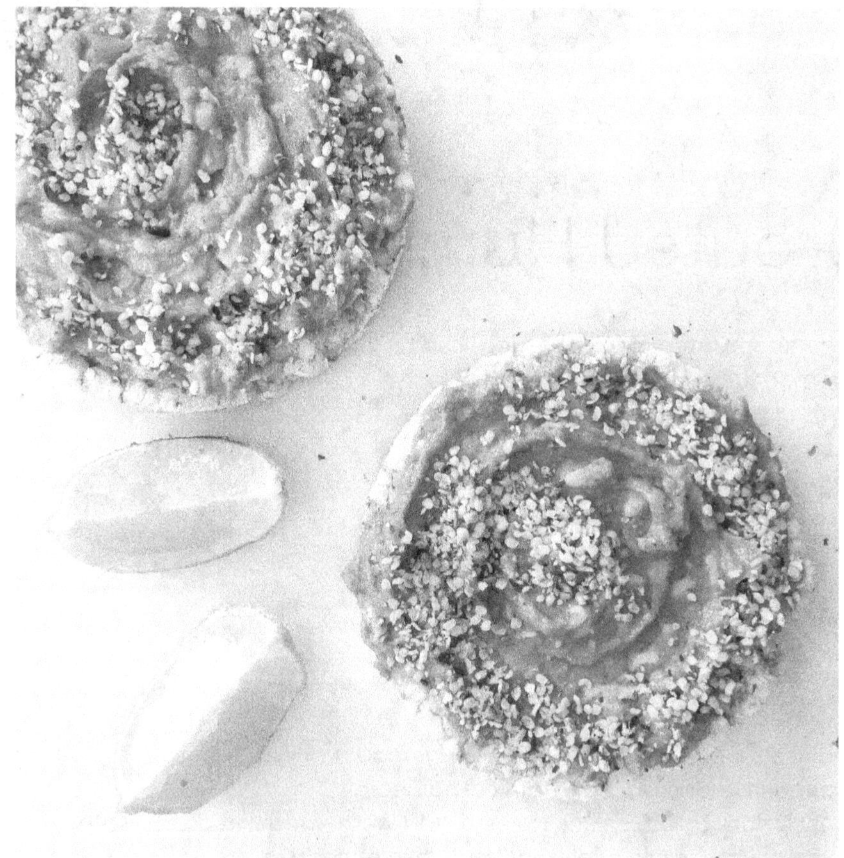

Guacamole

2 soft avocados
½ organic tomato
Handful cilantro
½ tsp sea salt
½ tsp garlic powder
¼ tsp black pepper
Dash cayenne pepper
Squeeze of lime juice

1. Cut avocados in half vertically and remove the seed. Scoop out insides and smash with a fork to reach desired consistency.
2. Dice tomato into small chunks and mince cilantro. Add both as well as the remainder of the ingredients to the avocado and press into mixture with a fork until combined. Best if used within a few hours.

<u>Snack ideas:</u>

Serve with plant based tacos (see recipe), spread on sandwich or wrap, use as a dip for raw veggies and pulp crackers, use as a dip for sweet potato fries (see recipe)

Mac n' Cheez Sauce

3 small gold potatoes
½ carrot
½ onion
2-3 cloves garlic
¾ c raw cashews
¼ c nutritional yeast
2 tbsp mustard
½-1 tsp white wine vinegar
½-1 tsp sea salt
½ tsp garlic powder
¼ tsp pepper
Dash cayenne pepper or paprika
Nut milk (I like unsweetened almond)

1. Soak cashews in water for at least 3 hours.
2. Peel and cut potatoes, carrots and onions and add to a pot of boiling water. Boil until tender, and keep the liquid broth they boiled in.
3. Put veggies, cashews, and spices into a high speed blender as well as about ½ c of the broth and ½ c almond milk. Blend on high for 2-3 minutes or until combined.
4. Taste mixture and add spices according to taste. I usually add more nutritional yeast, mustard or salt to get the taste I'm in the mood for! Add more or less liquid for desired consistency as well.

Meal ideas:

Serve over brown rice noodles or whole wheat noodles (elbows and fuseli are my favorite shape!), use as a "nacho cheese" with any mexican inspired dish, drizzle over burrito bowls (see recipe), use as dip for fresh and baked veggies, put in a whole wheat or corn tortilla to make a quesadilla.

Recipe inspired by original "cruelty free mac and 'cheese'" recipe by Laura Davis. www.laurasveganeats.blogspot.com . @laura.e.davis

This recipe is one of my favorites in the whole book! I LOVE mac and cheese. I used to eat 2 boxes at a time, multiple times a week in high school. I still eat this at least every week if not multiple. You don't have to give up your favorite foods to nourish your body. You just have to upgrade them! I hope you enjoy it. I found this recipe through a dear friend and modified to to my taste. Surround yourself with people who help you in this way, too!

Cashew Cream

1 c raw cashews (not roasted or salted)
2-3 cloves garlic
2 tbsp nutritional yeast
½ tsp sea salt
¼ tsp pepper
Almond milk

1. Soak cashews for at least 3 hours in water or overnight.

2. Add all ingredients to a high speed blender and blend on high for 2-3 minutes or until combined. Slowly add more almond milk to get desired consistency.
3. Taste and adjust spices according to taste.

<u>Meal ideas:</u>

Over spiralized zucchini noodles or pasta as an "alfredo" sauce, drizzled over a burrito or buddha bowl (see recipe), over mashed potatoes as creamy gravy, as a dip for crackers or veggies, as a base for a creamy soup, as a healthy alternative for anything that calls for heavy cream (if you remove spices), sour cream (add vinegar)

This sauce is a HUBBY favorite. It has become an absolute staple! If you want to introduce your family to healthier alternatives, start by upgrading to cashew cream and sharing it with loved ones in your recipes.

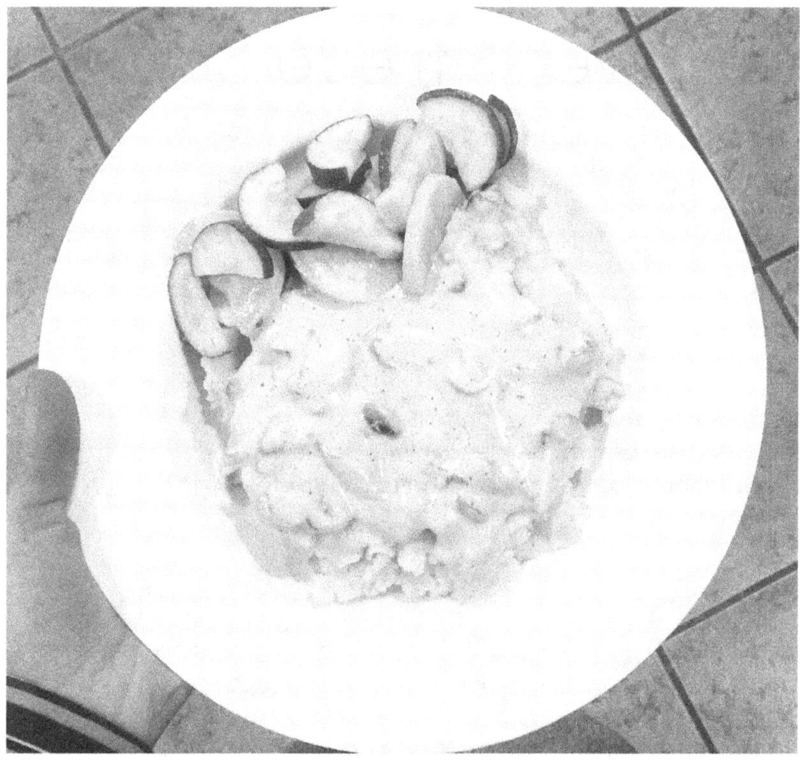

Creamy Mushroom Gravy

See my "cashew cream" recipe
1-2 c sliced mushrooms (any variety)

1. Make cashew cream according to its' recipe.
2. Slice mushrooms and saute them on medium-low until soft. Add cream sauce to the pan and stir with the mushrooms and their juices until combined.

<u>Meal ideas:</u>

Serve over a bowl of mashed potatoes and sauteed veggies, over pasta noodles for a plant based "stroganoff", use in place of "cream of mushroom soup" for any recipe.

Cauliflower Alfredo Sauce

See my "cashew cream" recipe
1.5 c of steamed cauliflower florets
1 tbsp nutritional yeast
1 tsp sea salt
Black pepper

1. Make cashew cream according to its' recipe.
2. Throw cauliflower into the blender with cashew sauce and add more garlic, salt, and nutritional yeast according to your taste. Blend on high until combined!

<u>Meal ideas:</u>

Serve over spiralized veggies or pasta as an "alfredo" sauce, serve as a creamy cauliflower soup, use as a dip for crackers or baked veggies

I'm a sucker for cheese, what can I say? Another favorite!

Thai Peanut Sauce

½ c natural peanut butter
2 tbsp organic (non gmo) tamari sauce (or soy sauce)
1 tbsp pure maple syrup
Dash cayenne pepper
Water

Add all ingredients to a bowl and whisk together. Slowly add more water to reach desired consistency.

Meal ideas:

Serve over rice and sauteed veggies for a stir-fry, use as a marinade for baked tofu, use as a dipping sauce for grilled veggie kabobs

Creamy Tahini Dressing

½ c tahini
2 tbsp stone ground mustard (with seeds)
1 tbsp fresh squeezed lemon juice
1 tbsp nutritional yeast
½ tsp sea salt
Pepper
Filtered water

Mix tahini with water until you reach desired consistency (thick or runny).
Add all other ingredients and mix until combined. Taste and add more ingredients to get the taste you like!
Store in the fridge. Dressing will harden so add a little water before serving.

Meal ideas:

Serve as a dressing over any salad (makes a great "ceasar" salad dressing), drizzle over a buddha bowl or burrito bowl, use as a dipping sauce for sweet potato fries or baked veggies

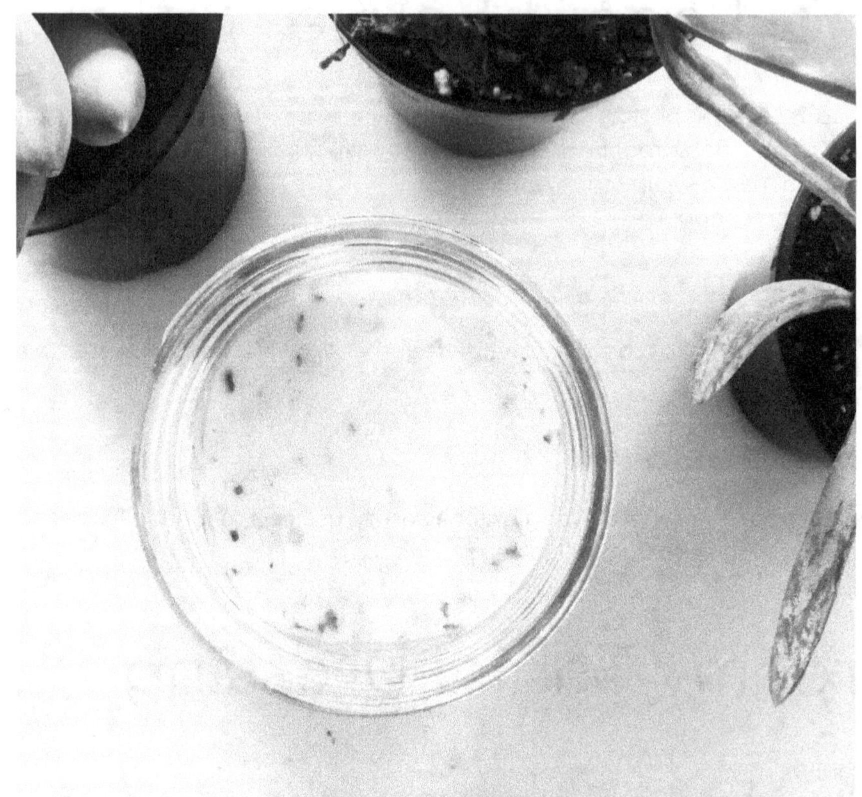

Almost Ranch Dressing

1 c unsweetened coconut yogurt
1 tbsp lemon juice (or 1 tsp white wine vinegar)
2 tsp nutritional yeast
¼ tsp fresh dill or spice
¼ tsp garlic powder
¼ tsp basil
¼ tsp parsley
¼ tsp black pepper

Add combine all ingredients in a bowl or blender and add more or less ingredients to achieve desired taste. Store in the fridge.

Serve over any salad, use as a dipping sauce for raw veggies, or a sauce for plant-based pizza

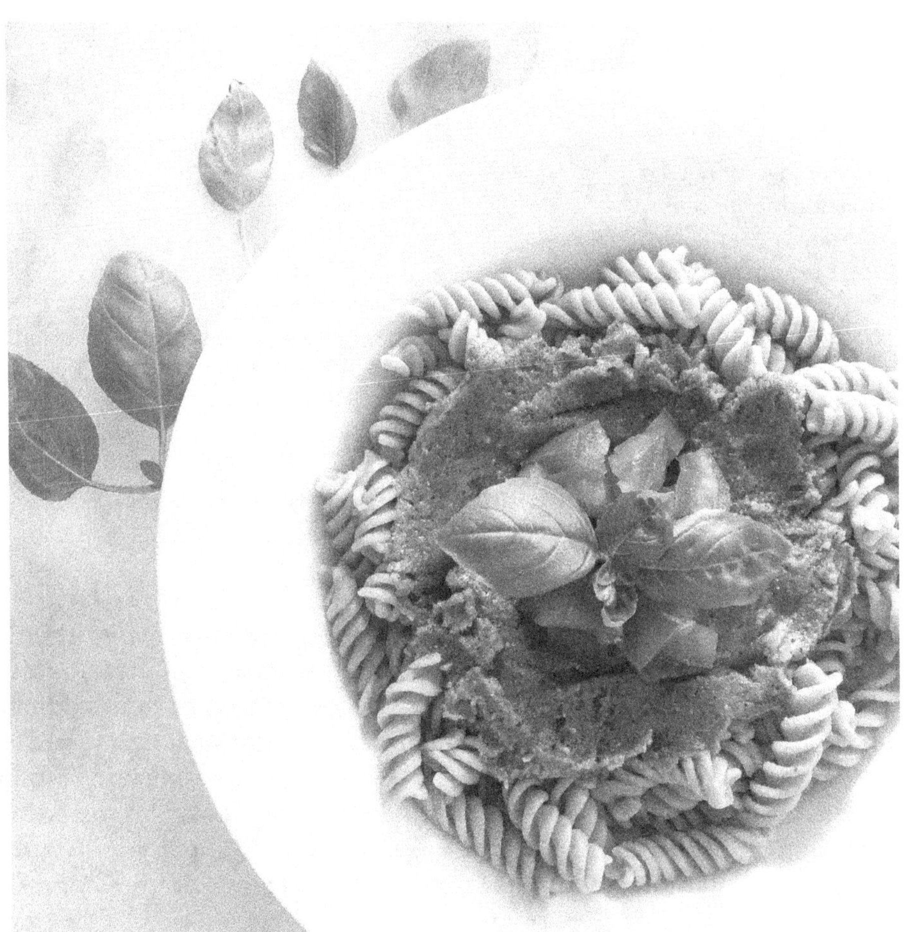

Spinach Pesto

1 c fresh basil
1/2 c fresh spinach
1/2 c pine nuts (or cashews)
1/4 c raw walnuts
3 cloves garlic, crushed
2-3 tbsp extra virgin olive oil

2 tbsp fresh lemon juice
2 tbsp nutritional yeast
1/2 tsp sea salt
1/2 tsp black pepper

Combine all ingredients in a food processor or high speed blender. Blend until desired consistency is reached, whether chunky or smooth.

<u>Meal ideas:</u>

Mixed into brown rice or quinoa pasta noodles, served over spiralized zucchini noodles, as a base for a veg pizza, as a dip for pulp crackers or raw veggies, as a spread on avocado toast or a sandwich/wrap

Spinach is a food you want to include in your diet each day (or other leafy greens!). Spinach is high in vitamin c, vitamin k, iron, calcium and folate. It is a great food for mama's trying for a baby or pregnant to provide vital nutrients to the fetus and prevent anemia. The vitamin k is also great for boosting the nutrients of a mother's breastmilk as newly born infants have naturally lower levels of vitamin k. Calcium is also important for nourishing a breastfeeding mother as this is one of the first nutrients to become deficient in. If you are a mama or want to be or know one - eat your spinach!

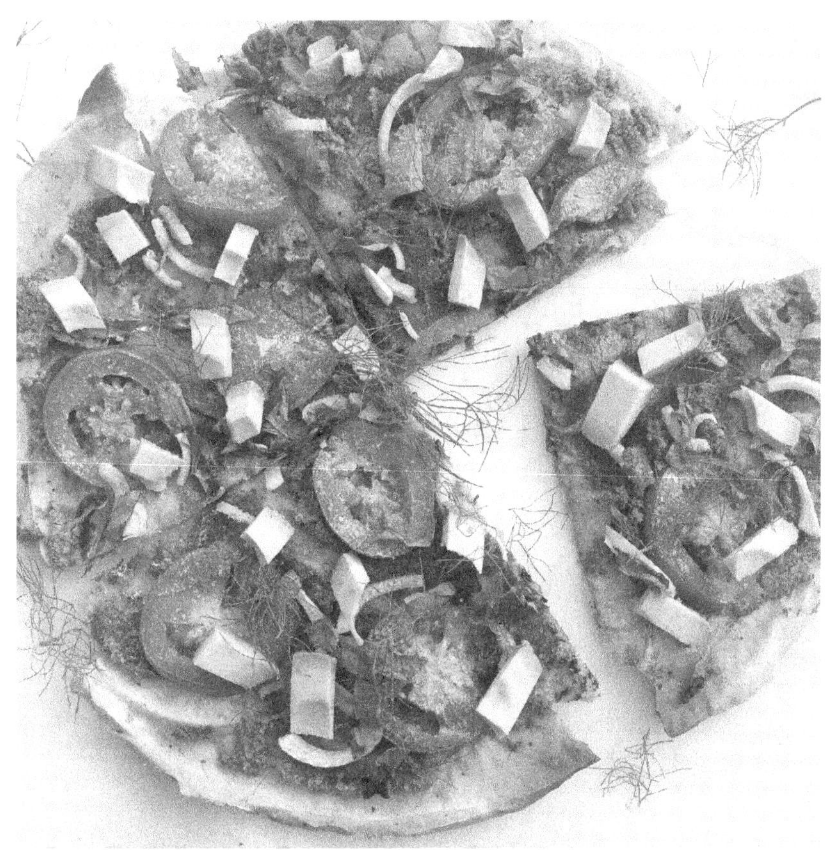

Cashew Parmesan

1 c raw cashews
1-2 tbsp nutritional yeast
1 tsp garlic powder
½ tsp sea salt
Pepper

Add ingredients into a blender and pulse mixture until you get a powdery/crumbly texture similar to parmesan cheese.

<u>Meal ideas:</u>

Sprinkle over plant-based pizza, stir into your favorite pasta sauce or sprinkle on top

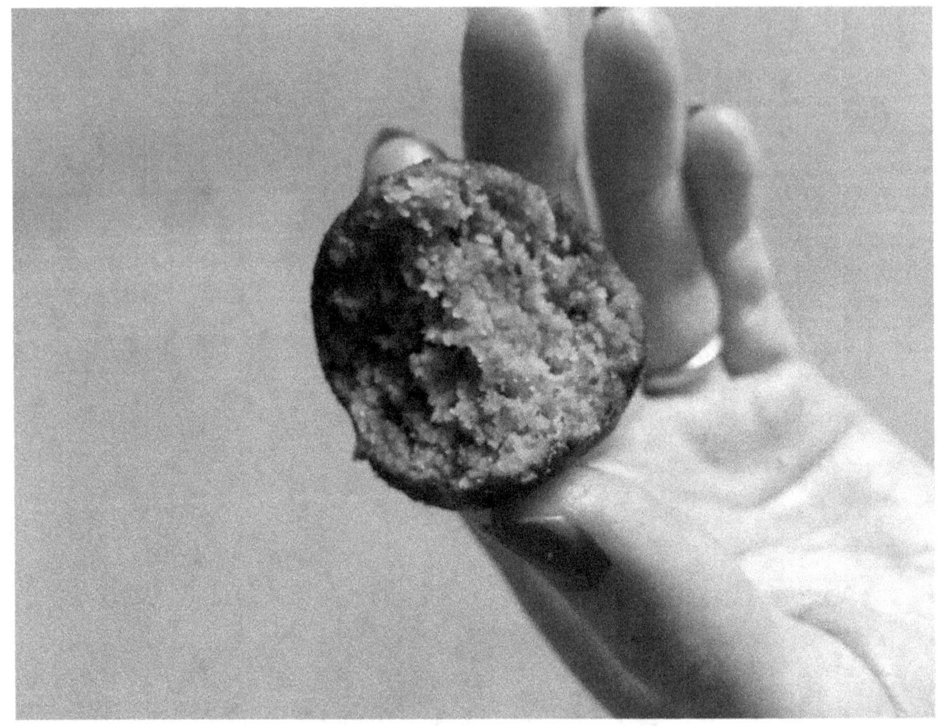

Coconut Berry Nice Cream

1 can organic full fat coconut milk
½ c frozen berries
1 tbsp maple syrup
Nut milk or water

1. Freeze can of coconut milk in an ice cube tray for at least 6 hours or overnight.
2. Add ice cubes to a high speed blender as well as maple syrup. Keep scraping down sides and blending and slowly add nut milk to get desired consistency. The less the better for more thickness.
3. Add berries and pulse blender for chunks or blend on high until combined, whatever you prefer!
4. Enjoy with some cacao nibs or fruit on top.

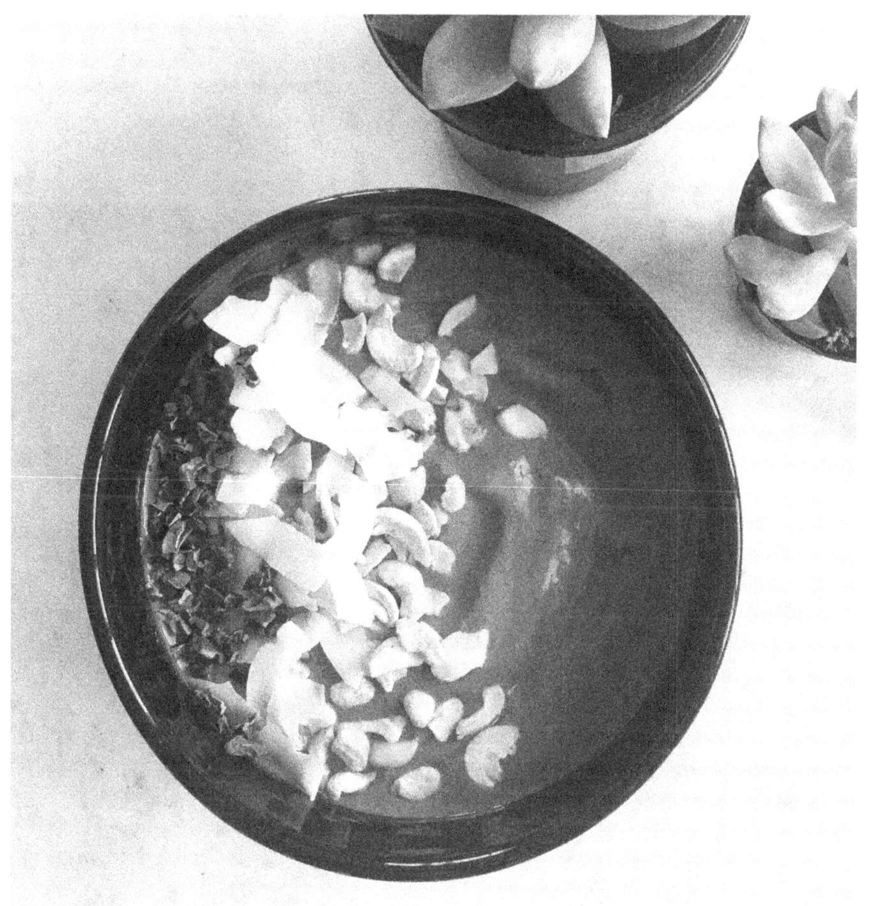

Chocolate Nice Cream

3-4 frozen bananas
2 tbsp raw cacao powder
1 tbsp maple syrup
1 c nut mlk

1. Add all ingredients in a high speed blender and blend for 1-3 minutes or until completely combined. Add nut milk slowly to get desired consistency, stopping blender to scrape down sides if necessary. The thicker the better!
2. Serve with fresh fruit on top.

Add any frozen fruit of choice or remove chocolate for variations! Recipe is versatile so play with it, leaving the bananas as the base for the nice cream.

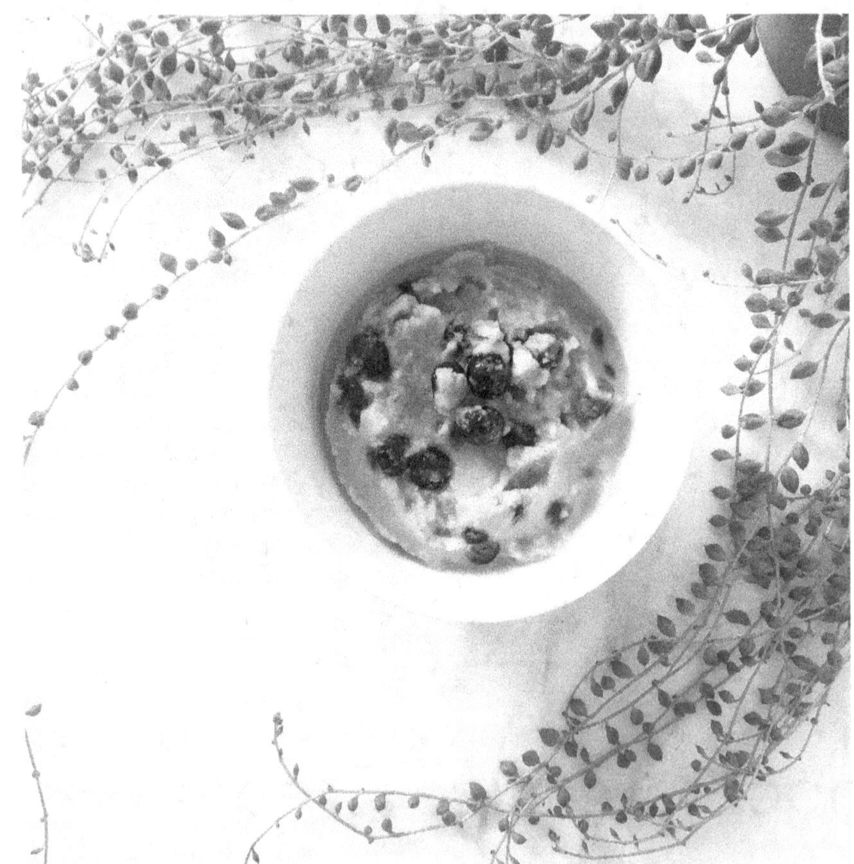

1 Minute Nice Cream

1 c frozen wild blueberries (the smaller the better)
1-2 c nut milk
1 tsp maple syrup or raw honey

1. Place frozen blueberries into a bowl. Pour nut milk over blueberries ⅓ c at a time and stir mixture. Blueberries will begin to freeze the nut milk. Add more

or less milk for desired consistency. GIve the mixture time to freeze up. Drizzle with sweetner at the end, and enjoy!

This was the first healthy treat I ever made. I got the recipe when I was serving as a missionary for my church, through the grapevine! It was the first time I realized that desserts could be healthy and that I could fully enjoy them without feeling sluggish or regretful afterwards.

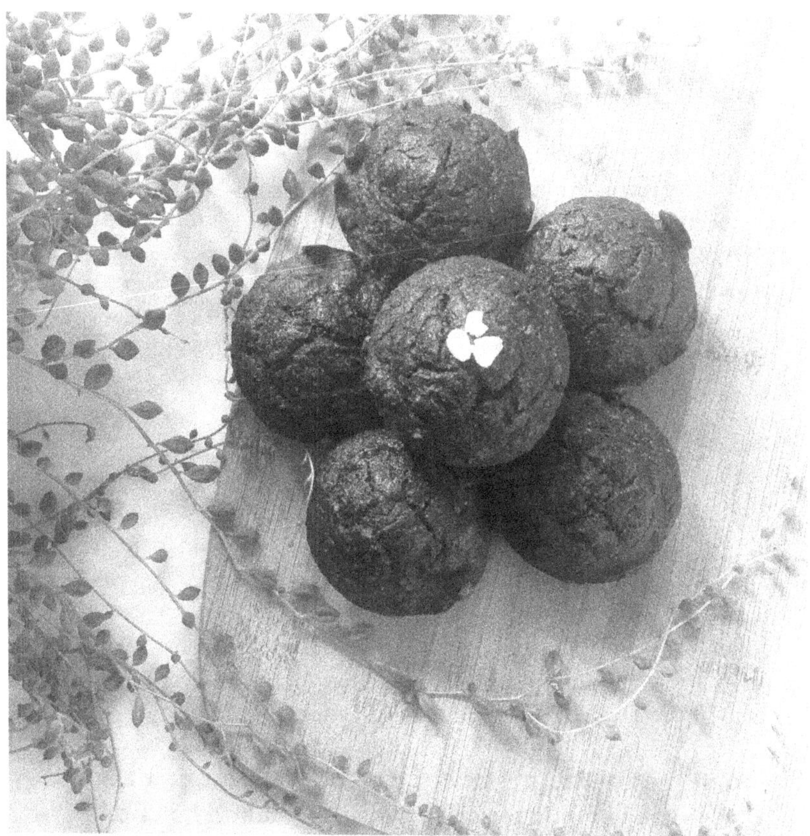

Raw Cacao Muffins

3 ripe bananas
1 1/2 c traditional rolled oats
3/4 c almond pulp (or almond flour)
1 flax egg (1 tbsp flax meal + 3 tbsp water & soak 5 mins)

1/2 c raw cacao powder (or unsweetened cocoa)
2 tbsp pure maple syrup
1/4 c coconut sugar
1/4 c coconut oil, melted
1 tsp vanilla extract
1 tsp baking powder
1/2 tsp baking soda
1/4 tsp sea salt
1/2 c cacao nibs, carob chips, or semi-sweet choc chips

1. Preheat oven to 350 degrees F. Grease a muffin tin with coconut oil or line with muffin cups. Whip up the flax egg and allow it to sit while you prepare the remainder of the muffin batch.
2. Put all ingredients (except choc chips) into a high-speed blender. Blend until smooth, but try not to over-blend. I did about 1 min, then scrape the sides, 1 more minute.
3. If you don't have a high-speed blender, then smash bananas in a bowl and add all wet ingredients to it. Combine. Once combined, add all dry ingredients and mix again. You will need to use oat flour instead of oats, OR make sure to blend up your oats in a food processor/blender beforehand to make oat flour.
4. Spoon batter equally into the muffin tins. Sprinkle your chocolate chips on top!
5. Cook in the oven for 25-30 minutes. Remove from oven and allow to cool for 30 minutes before serving.

Treat ideas:

Add homemade nut butter spread on top, broken and sprinkled over your nice cream, as a fun breakfast with nut milk to wash it down, as a baked good for a good friend

Cacao is one of the earth's most magical foods! Although the industry has added sugar, butter and other chemicals and called it "chocolate", cacao in its original form is actually a very healthy and beneficial food. It serves as a natural source of energy for some with its trace amounts of naturally occurring caffeine, while also having a calming effect with it's source of magnesium. I have used it as a morning boost or enjoyed it's calming effects in the evening. It is also contains a small amount of healthy fats. Enjoy this rich, bitter, and diverse food and upgrade your chocolate cravings with cacao!

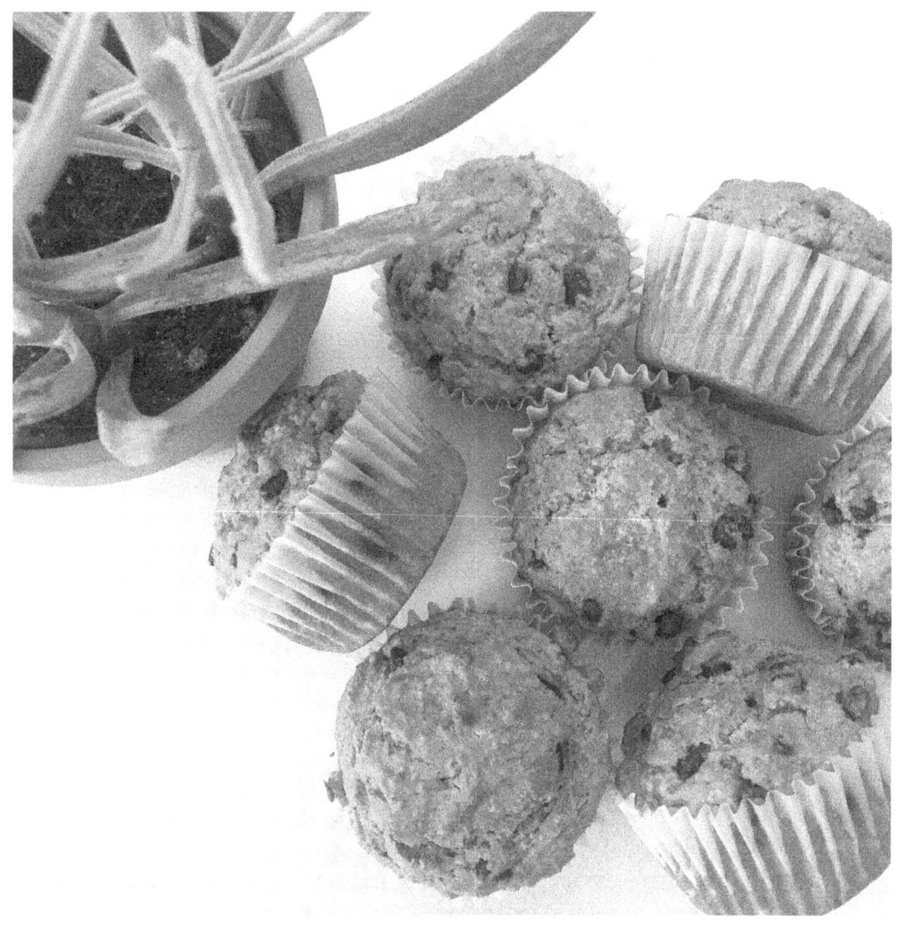

Veggie Muffins

1 c gluten-free or whole wheat baking flour
1 c rolled oats, ground into flour
1/2 c almond flour
2 tbsp flax meal
1 tsp baking soda
1 tsp baking powder
1 tsp ginger
1 tsp cinnamon
1/4 tsp nutmeg

1/4 tsp clove
1/4 tsp sea salt
1/2 - 1 c fresh grated carrot or zucchini
1 flax egg (or egg)
1 c nut milk
1/4 c pure maple syrup
2 tbsp olive oil
2 tsp pure vanilla extract
1/2 c dairy-free chocolate chips, nuts or dried fruit

** to make oat flour, simply grind rolled oats in a blender, magic bullet or food processor, I usually just "pulse" it so that it has small chunks of oats for a more fibrous consistency.

1. Preheat oven to 400 degrees and line muffin tin with paper muffin cups.
2. Combine all dry ingredients. Add grated veggies and combine. In a separate bowl, combine all wet ingredients. Add dry ingredients and wet ingredients together and mix until combined. Stir in chocolate chips.
3. Scoop batter into muffin tin, equally. Bake muffins for 25-30 minutes, or until golden brown and toothpick inserted leaves the muffin clean.
4. Remove muffin pan and allow to cool for 20 minutes before consuming. Good in the fridge for 5-7 days or in the freezer for 1 month.

<u>Treat ideas:</u>

This is a toddler favorite! Sneak some veggies in for picky kids. Freeze batches ahead of time and thaw or lunch boxes or "on the go".

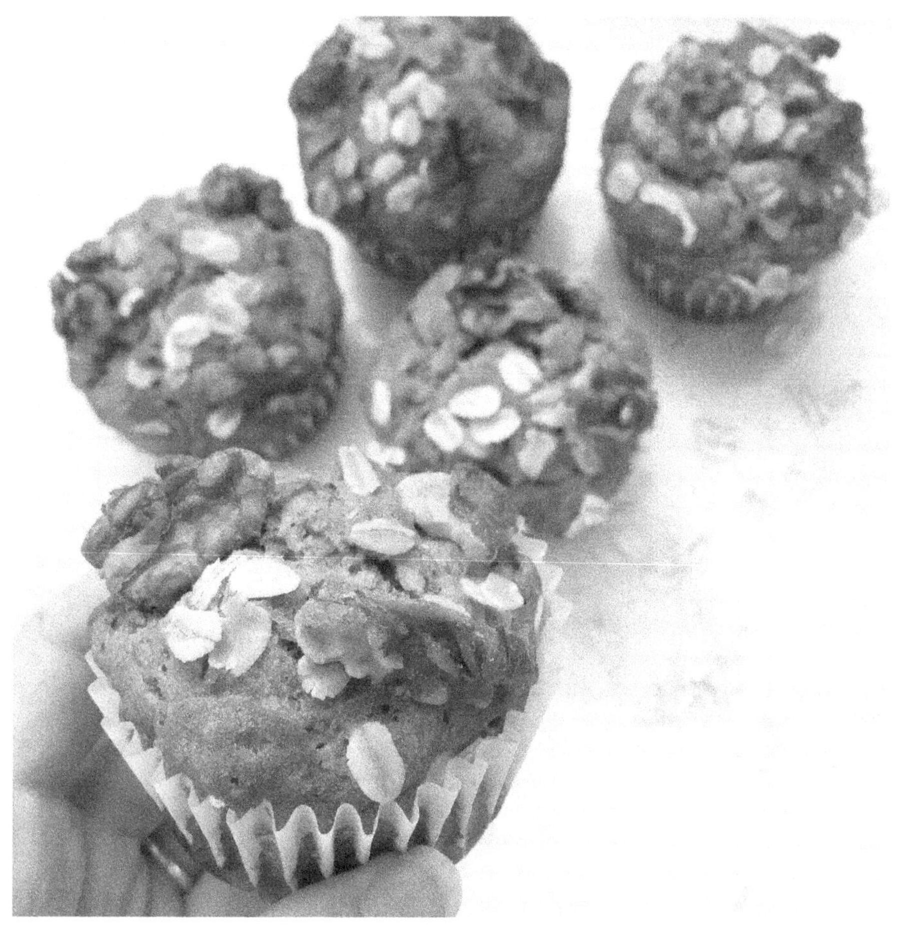

Good Ol' Banana Muffins

3 medium-large brown bananas
2 c gluten free or whole wheat baking flour
1 c rolled or instant oats
2 flax eggs (or eggs)
1/2 c coconut sugar
1/3 c unsweetened apple sauce (optional)
1/3 c coconut oil, melted
1-2 tablespoons pure maple syrup
1 tsp vanilla extract
1 tsp baking powder
1 tsp baking soda

1 tsp cinnamon
1/2 tsp nutmeg
1/2 tsp sea salt

1. Preheat oven to 375 degrees and line a muffin tin with paper muffin cups.
2. Mash bananas with a fork and then use a hand mixer to liquify. Add other wet ingredients and mix until combined.
3. Add all dry ingredients in another bowl, then add to wet ingredients and mix until combined.
4. The mixture will be thick! Add more oats/flour if too runny. Fill muffin tins equally.
5. Bake for 20 minutes or until toothpick comes out clean. Makes 12 muffins.

Treat ideas:

Breakfast muffins with nut butter or homemade raspberry jam spread on top.

I used this recipe to make Shilos birthday "cake" for his first birthday. I loved that it was sweet but had healthy clean ingredients.

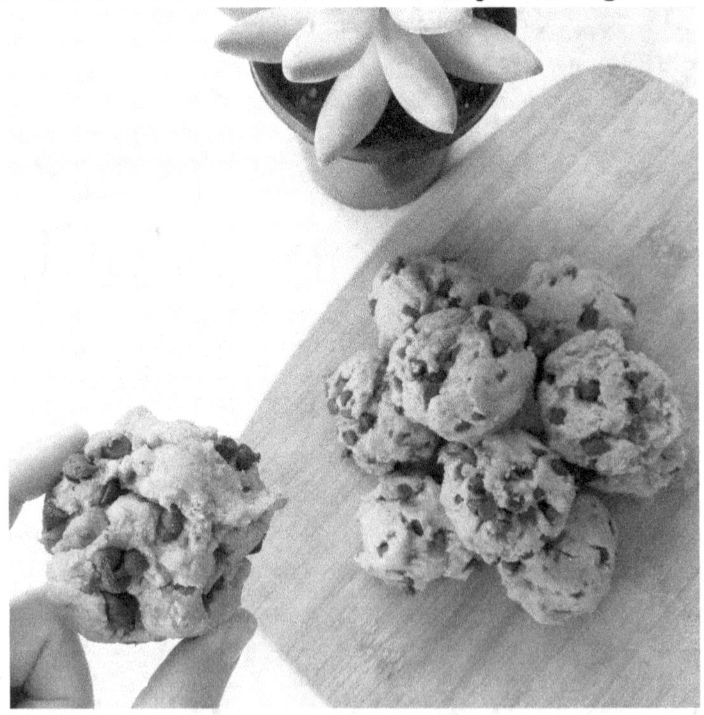

Pumpkin Spice Cookies

1 c 100% pure organic pumpkin
1 egg (or flax egg)
1/2 c coconut oil
1/2 c maple syrup
1 tsp vanilla
1 tsp almond milk
1 tsp baking soda
2 tsp baking powder
2 tsp cinnamon
1 tsp pumpkin spice (or 1 more tsp of cinnamon if you don't have this)
1/2 tsp sea salt
A dash of nutmeg, clove, and ginger
2 c Gluten-free or whole wheat baking flour
1/2 c Dairy-free chocolate chips

1. Preheat oven to 350 degrees F. Prepare a baking sheet covered in parchment paper.
2. Put coconut oil in a sauce pan and melt until liquid. Add honey if not already liquid. Combine oil, honey, pumpkin, vanilla & egg in a small bowl.
    a. If pumpkin and egg are not room temperature, coconut oil may harden again. Keep this in mind. You can warm the pumpkin slightly before adding to mixture and adding egg last.
3. In a separate bowl, combine baking soda & almond milk. Stir into pumpkin mixture.
4. In a large bowl, combine flour and other dried ingredients.. Once combined, add to pumpkin mixture - try not to over mix.
5. Fold in chocolate chips!
6. Using a spoon, scoop out cookies to about 1.5-2 in in diameter, and place on baking sheet. Space equally apart.
7. Bake for 12-15 minutes or until a toothpick comes out clean!

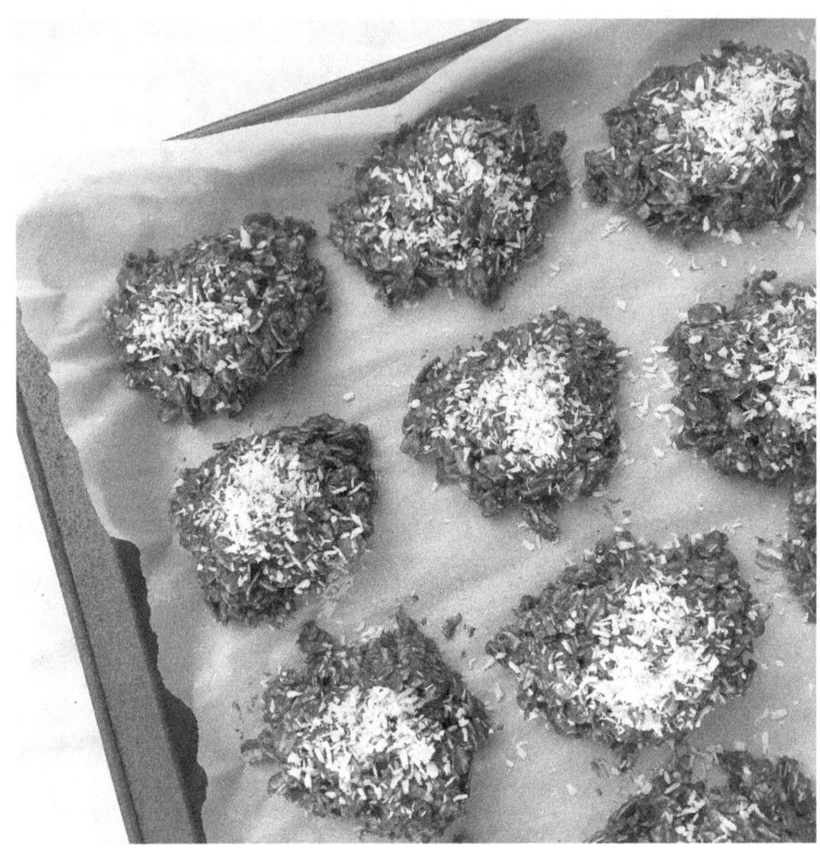

Almond Joy No-Bakes

4 c traditional rolled oats
½ c almond butter
½ c unsweetened coconut shreds (or coconut pulp)
½ c maple syrup
½ c coconut oil
6 tbsp cacao powder
2 tsp vanilla extract
½ tsp sea salt

1. Prepare a baking sheet with parchment paper. Put all ingredients in a bowl and use your hands to massage them together until combined.
2. Use a spoon and put 3-4" dollops onto the baking sheet, flatten if desired. Sprinkle with more coconut shreds on top.

3. Freeze for 3-4 hours. Try not to eat them all at once! They are addicting.

Modified from Melissa Chappells book FAVES
Find more of her recipes at @freshmelissa on Instagram or
www.freshmelissa.com

The original creator of the base of this recipe was my midwife for Arlo's birth, Melissa. I remember she brought me a box of these during one of our visits and I ate the whole thing in one sitting! I made her recipe and several variations of it throughout my pregnancy and it was a staple snack for me when I had a sugar craving. This is a great, healthy alternative if you need something to snack on!

Avocado Mousse

2 soft avocados
2-4 tbsp cacao powder
2 tbsp maple syrup
Nut milk

1. Put avocados, cacao and maple syrup in the blender and blend until combined. Add nut milk as needed to get desired consistency.
2. Refrigerate for at least 30 minutes and serve with strawberries on top.

Treat ideas:

Use as a healthy chocolate spread on toast/muffins, serve as chocolate sauce over nice cream, or enjoy alone with fruit on top.

Avocado is one of the richest plant based sources of healthy fats! Fats nourish the brain, the skin, the gut, and our hormones. Avocados closely resemble a mother's womb in it's appearance and function. This is no surprise, as the avocado is a very nourishing food for a woman. It's very essence is nurturing, and when we eat it, it nurtures and balances our hormones, reproductive organs, and thyroid. I try to eat some avocado every single day. You will find many recipes in this book to help you

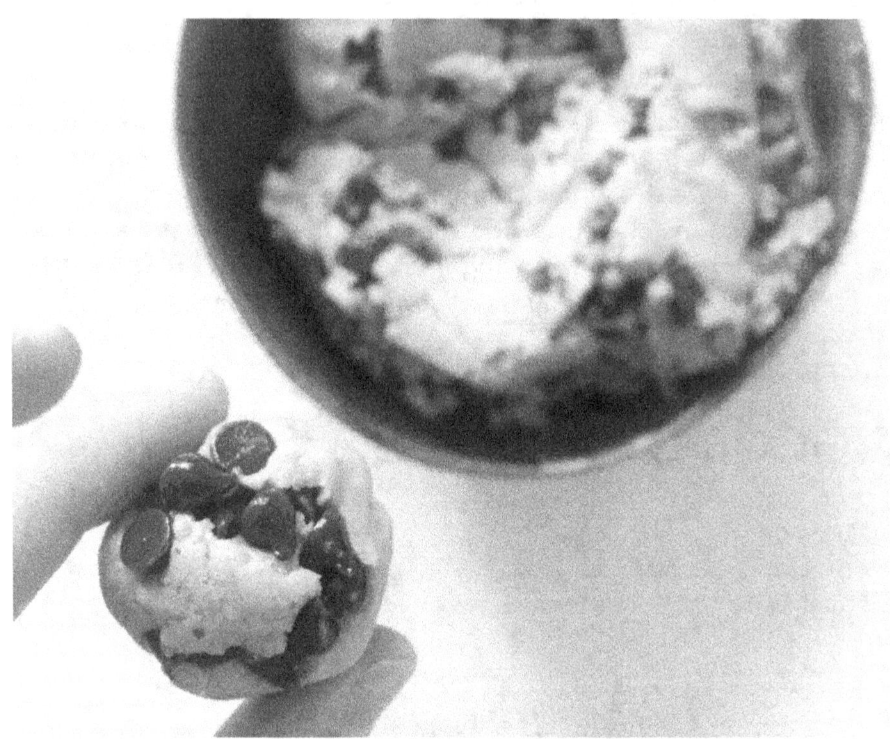

Nut Pulp Cookie Dough

1 c nut milk pulp (almond/cashew)
3/4 c raw almonds
2 tbsp nut butter
3 dates, chopped
1 tbsp raw honey or maple syrup
1/2 tsp ceylon cinnamon
1/2 tsp vanilla extract
pinch sea salt
nut milk (as needed) to help blend
1/2 c dairy free chocolate chips

Options:

Sub out nut milk pulp for almond flour or coconut flour, add more nut milk if dry.

1. Put all ingredients together into a food processor or blender, except for the chocolate chips and nut milk.
2. Blend all ingredients together, adding 1/2 tsp of nut milk at a time as needed to help it blend together. Be careful not to add too much!
3. Once blended well, mix in chocolate chips with a spoon.
4. Spoon out bite sized portions and roll them in a ball, placing them into a container. Freeze bites for 2-3 hours before serving for hard consistency, refrigerate for softer bites.

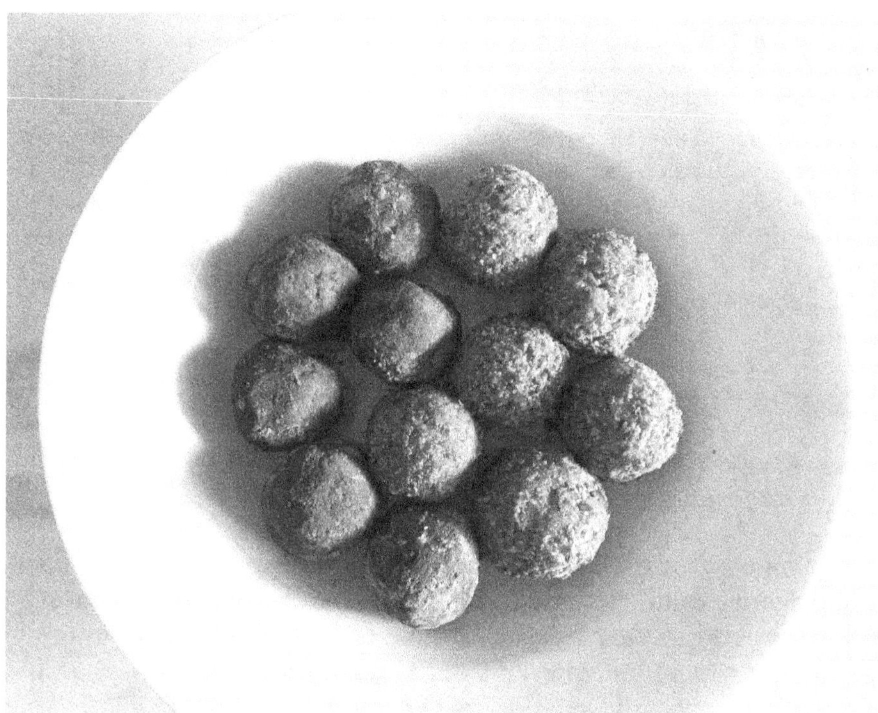

"Baby Moon" Bites

1.5 c coconut milk pulp
1 c almond butter
½ c raw honey
Cinnamon

Cacao powder
Ground flax seed

Options:
Sub coconut milk pulp with coconut flour or shredded coconut. Add nut milk as needed for consistency.

1. Add coconut milk pulp (or shredded coconut that has been ground to smaller pieces - you can pulse in your blender), almond butter and honey into a bowl and use hands to mix together thoroughly.
2. Roll into 2" balls and then roll balls in cinnamon, cacao or ground flaxseed to cover the outside. Place baby moon bites onto a baking sheet with parchment paper or into a glass container and refrigerate or freeze for 2-3 hours before serving.

<u>Treat ideas:</u>

These are a great healthy snack for little ones! If you freeze them into smaller balls they are good for on-the-go. I make them about ½" size bites for him.

My Shilo named these his "baby moon bites" because we often use names of his favorite things for healthy foods so that he grows an interest and fondness in them. He has always loved the moon and so anything that resembles a circle (and when bitten, a crescent) becomes a "moon". This is a healthy alternative to fruit snacks and other similar junk treats out there.

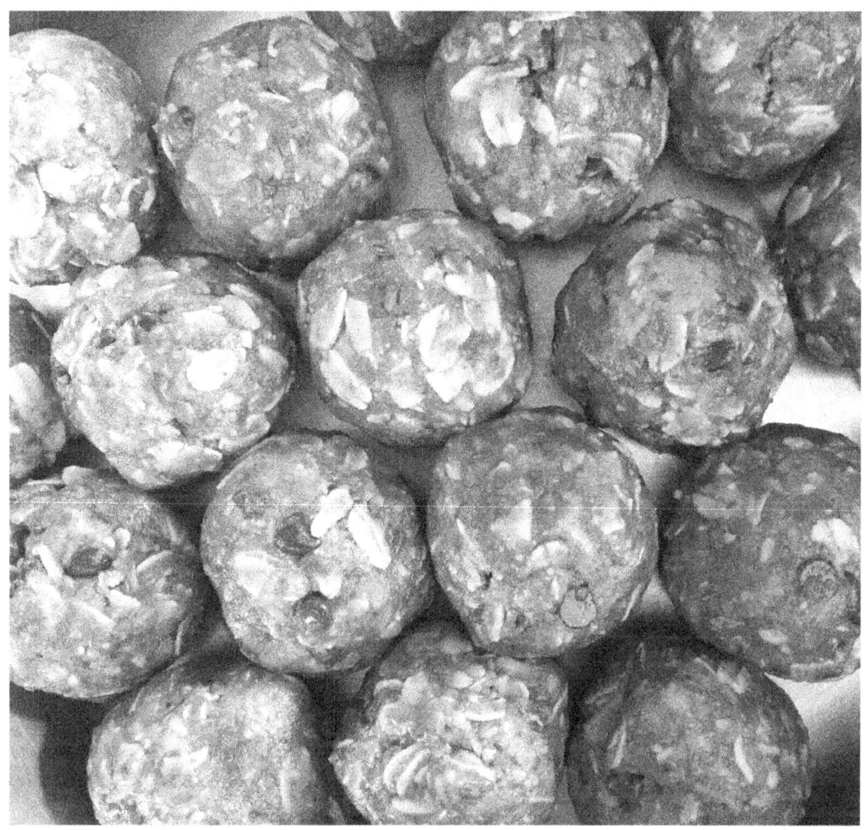

Power Seed Bites

1 c rolled or instant oats
1 - 1.5 c nut butter
½ c raw honey
1 tbsp chia seeds
1 tbsp flax seeds
1 tbsp sunflower seeds
1 tbsp hemp seeds
Pinch sea salt
Cinnamon

1. Combine all ingredients in a bowl and use hands to combine. Add more nut butter or honey as necessary to help bites stay together.

2. Roll into 2" balls and then roll balls in cinnamon or more seeds (if desired) to cover the outside. Place power seed bites onto a baking sheet with parchment paper or into a glass container and refrigerate or freeze for 2-3 hours before serving.

Cheezy Popcorn

2 c air popped or plain popcorn (not microwave)
1 tbsp melted coconut oil
2 tbsp nutritional yeast
1 tsp pink himalayan sea salt

1. Add popcorn to large bowl and drizzle melted coconut oil over it. Mix with a spoon until popcorn is covered. Sprinkle nutritional yeast and salt over popcorn and continue to stir until combined.
2. Add more nutritional yeast for more "cheezy" flavor. Serve warm.

Microwaveable popcorn contains harmful chemicals in the lining of the bags that are damaging to your health. They also are often full of butter o inflammatory oils and a frightening amount of salt. Consider air popped and enjoy this recipe as an alternative!

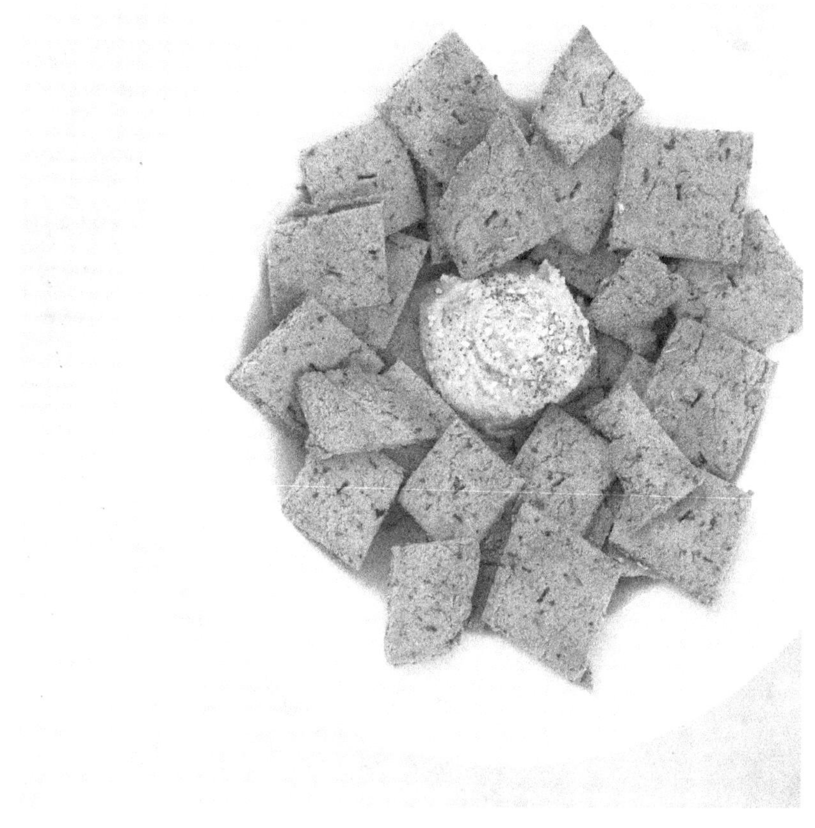

Pulp Crackers

1 c almond or cashew pulp (or almond flour)
3 tbsp ground flax seed
2 tbsp nutritional yeast
½ tsp garlic powder
½ tsp sea salt
Pepper
Filtered water

Optional spices/additions:
Rosemary, basil, oregano, chia seeds, sunflower seeds

1. Preheat oven to 400 degrees. Prepare a baking sheet with parchment paper.

2. Mix pulp with ground flax and spices until combined. Notice the consistency of the mixture and if necessary add a little bit of water at a time until you get a "dough".
3. Spread mixture evenly on a baking sheet covered in parchment paper until it is very thin. Aim for less than ¼ inch. The thinner, the crispier!
4. Score the mixture with a pizza cutter to achieve cracker shaped squares. Around 2" by 2" is good. Sprinkle with more nutritional yeast.
5. Place sheet in oven for 40 minutes, flipping halfway. Cook longer if edges are not browned. Place under broiler for 2-3 minutes at the end to get more crisp.

<u>Meal ideas:</u>

Serve dipped in guacamole or hummus, served with vegetarian chili (see recipe)

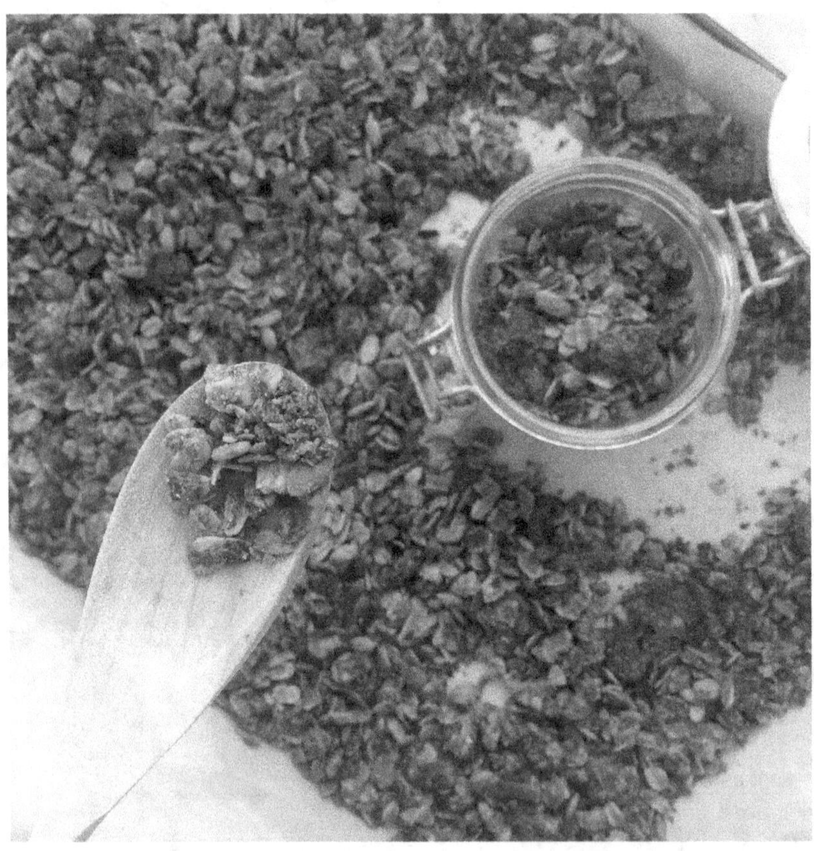

Earthy Granola

1.5 c rolled oats
½ c unsweetened coconut shreds
½ c sliced almonds
½ c chopped walnuts
½ c pumpkin seeds
½ c sunflower seeds
¼ c chia seeds
¼ c flax seeds
¼ c hemp seeds
¼ c cacao nibs
⅓ c coconut oil, melted
½ c nut butter
¼ c maple syrup
6 dates chopped
2 tbsp ceylon cinnamon
1 tbsp vanilla extract
½ tsp sea salt

1. Preheat oven to 275 degrees. Prepare baking sheet with parchment paper and set aside.
2. In a large mixing bowl, add all dry ingredients and stir until combined.
3. In a separate small pan, melt coconut oil and then whisk in nut butter, maple syrup and vanilla until combined.
4. Pour wet mixture into dry mixture and stir until all dry ingredients are covered and mixture is completely combined.
5. Spread evenly on the baking sheet and bake for 45 minutes, stirring mixture every 15 minutes or so. Broil on high for 1-2 minutes at the end if necessary for desired crisp!
6. Allow to cool before storing in an airtight container.

<u>Meal ideas:</u>

Eat with coconut yogurt and fruit, sprinkle over a smoothie bowl or nice cream, enjoy with nut milk, warm up apples or peaches over the stove with coconut milk and cinnamon and sprinkle granola on top for a healthy "crisp" or "cobbler" feel.

If you really want to feel granola…. Try this recipe! Just make sure you eat it in the wilderness and don't shave your armpits either. This recipe is extremely nutrient dense as it contains several nuts and seeds making it a wonderful source of plant protein, healthy fats, and natural sugars as well. Walnuts very closely resemble the human brain… They are also very nourishing for the brain! Walnuts are high in omega-3 fatty acids which support brain health and in turn mental health.

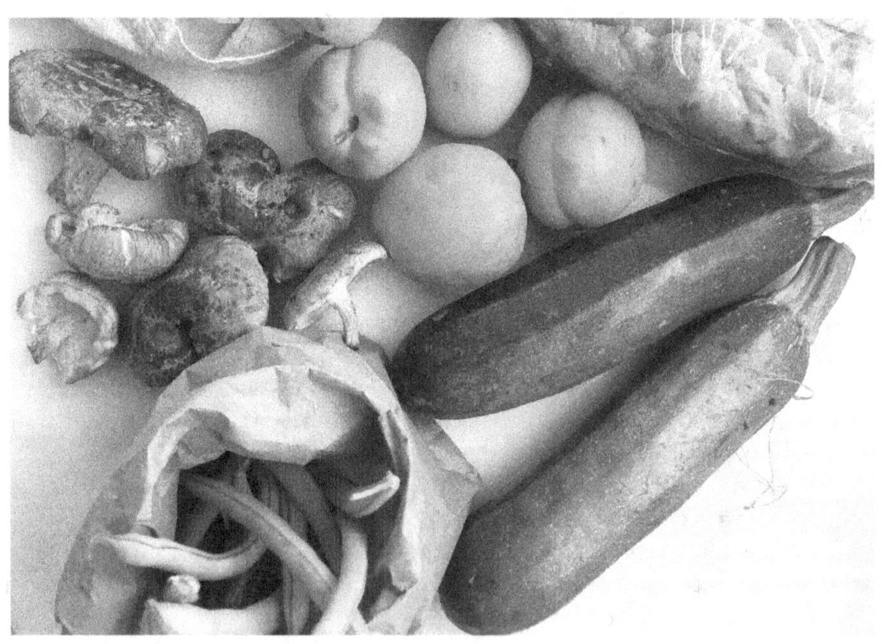

SIDES / BREADS

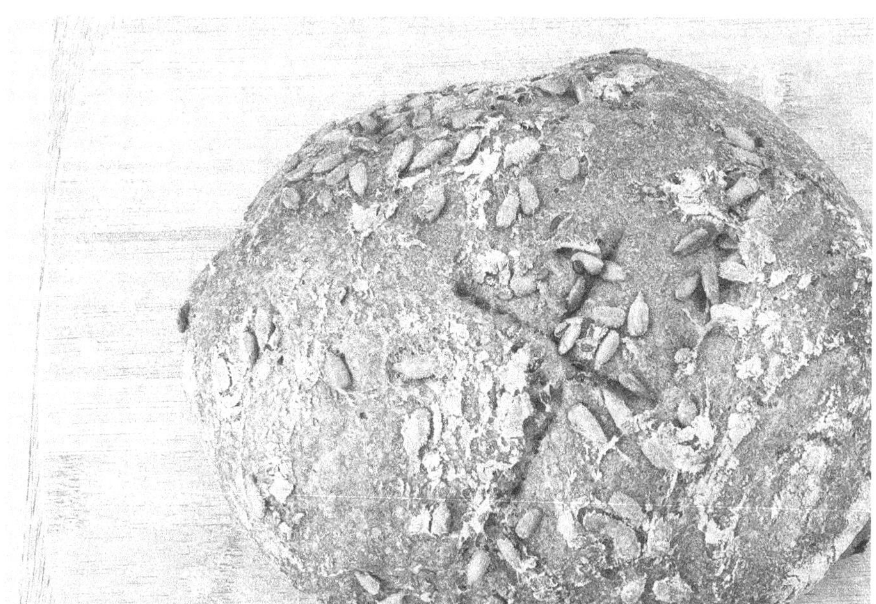

Whole Wheat and Seed Artisan Bread

3 c whole wheat all purpose flour
1 tsp sea salt
½ tsp active yeast
1.5 c warm water
¼ c sunflower seeds
⅛ c flax seeds

1. Add yeast and warm water to a bowl and whisk for a minute until dissolved.
2. Add flour and salt and stir until combined. Roll dough in sunflower and flax seeds and sprinkle until desired amount sticks to the outside.
3. Cover with plastic wrap and allow to sit at room temperature overnight or for 24 hours.
4. Turn dough on to a well floured surface and carefully shape into a ball. Allow to rest for 30 minutes.
5. Preheat oven to 450 degrees. Place a baking dish or bread dish into the oven while preheating.

6. Carefully transfer bread to baking dish, sprinkle with additional seeds if desired and slash an "x" on top of the loaf. Cover and bake for 30 minutes.
7. Uncover and bake for an additional 10-15 minutes or until golden brown.
8. Allow to cool completely before slicing.

<u>Serving ideas:</u>

Avocado toast, with homemade raspberry chia jam and nut butter, on the side of soup

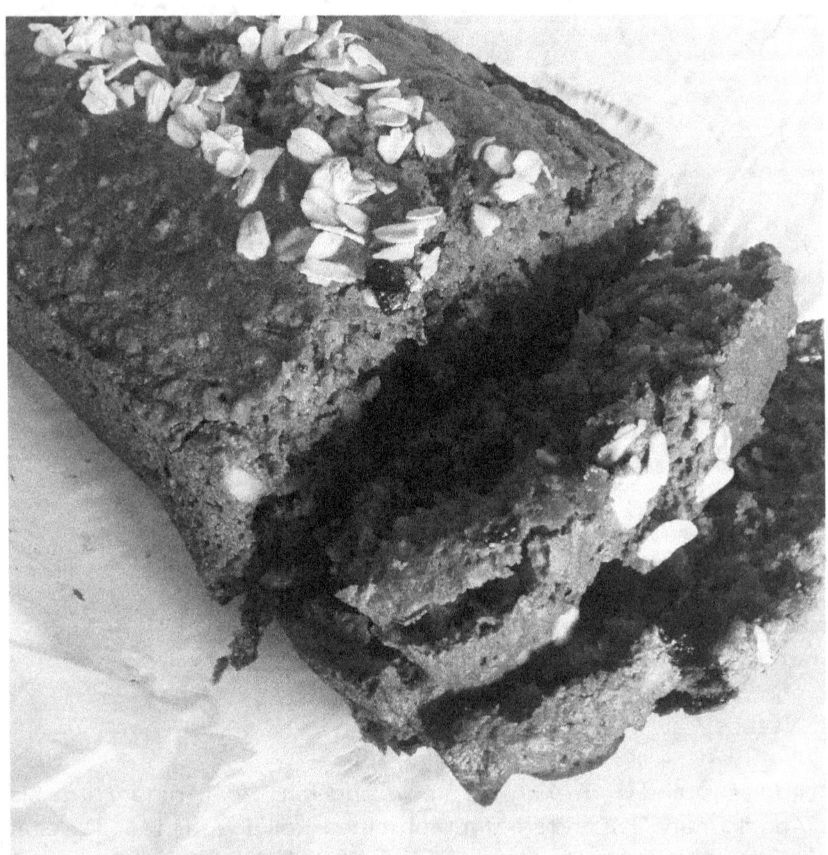

Zucchini Bread

1 c gluten free or whole wheat baking flour
1 c rolled or instant oats
2 c grated zucchini

1 c coconut sugar
⅓ c coconut oil, melted
¼ c applesauce
2 flax eggs (or organic eggs)
2 tsp vanilla extract
1 tbsp ceylon cinnamon
½ tsp baking powder
½ tsp baking soda
¼ tsp sea salt
½-1 c of fruit or nuts
(I like blueberries, walnuts, or dairy free chocolate chips)

1. Preheat oven to 400 degrees. Line a bread pan with parchment paper.
2. Mix dry ingredients until combined. In a separate bowl combine wet ingredients. Add zucchini to dry ingredients first and then add wet ingredient mixture and stir until combined.
3. Pour mixture into bread pan and sprinkle with rolled oats on top. Bake for about 1 hour, or until toothpick comes out clean and outside is browned.
4. Allow to sit and cool for 30 minutes before slicing.

<u>Serving ideas:</u>

Spread raspberry chia jam or nut butter on top, eat as a healthy breakfast, give to a toddler to sneak in some veggies

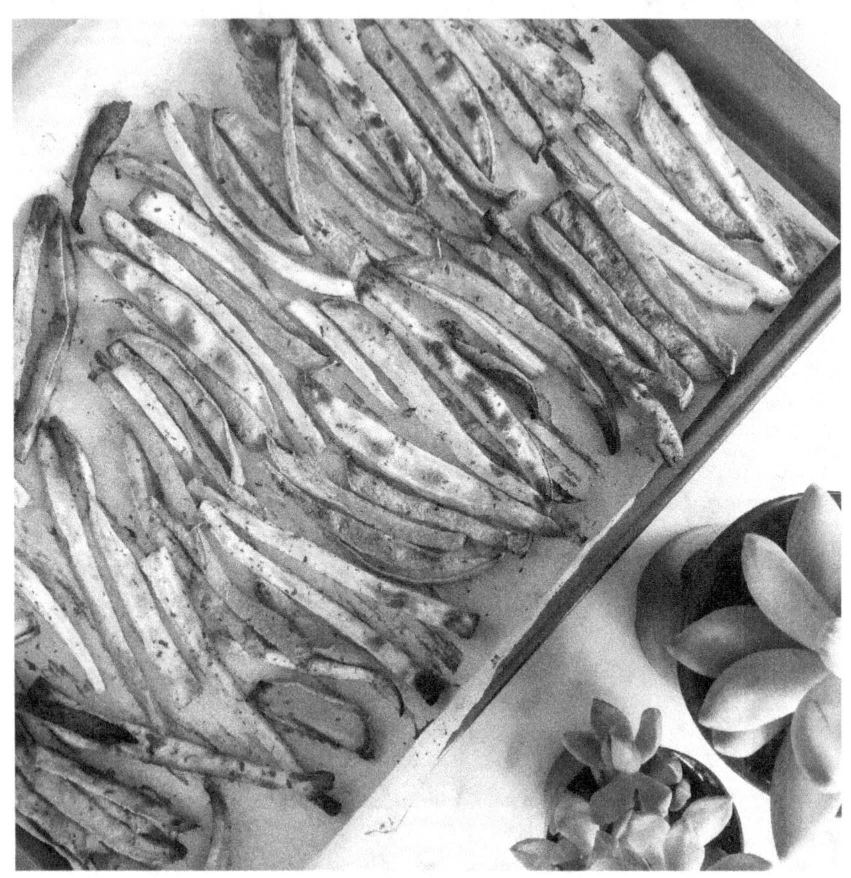

Sweet Potato Fries

3 large sweet potatoes
1 tbsp avocado oil
Sea salt
Pepper
Cayenne pepper

1. Preheat oven to 400 degrees. Cover baking sheet in parchment paper.
2. Cut up sweet potatoes in long, thin strips (to closely resemble fries). About ½ inch in thickness.
3. Put potato fries in a baggie and pour oil and spices over them. Mix and shake in bag until fully covered.

4. Spread evenly on baking sheet. Bake for 30-45 minutes, flipping halfway.

<u>Serving ideas:</u>

Dip in fresh guacamole, on the side of black bean burgers, spice with maple syrup and cinnamon instead to make a treat.

The sweet potato is a very nutrient dense foods. It contains an antioxidant called beta-carotene that is a great anti-inflammatory. It is rich in vitamins b, vitamin c, vitamin e, vitamin k and minerals like phosphorus, calcium, and iron. It is a healthy carbohydrate meaning that it is a great source of energy for the body. It is also high in fiber and therefore helps to improve overall digestion. Like my dad says after every Thanksgiving - "they are pretty 'yam' good."

Caprese Salad

1 english cucumber
1-2 heirloom tomato
1 c vegan mozzarella (or normal)
Olive oil
Balsamic vinegar
Sea salt
Pepper

Cut cucumber, tomato and mozzarella into 1 inch chunks. Mix together in a bowl and drizzle with olive oil and vinegar. Spice according to your taste and enjoy!

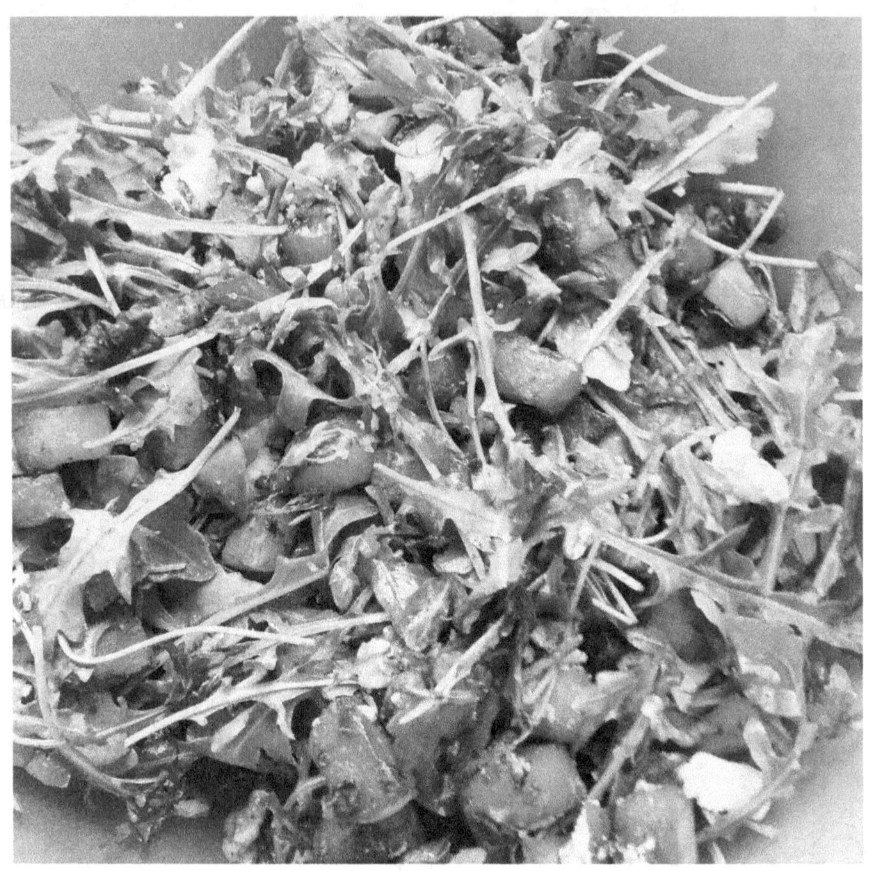

Maple Butternut Hash

1 medium butternut squash
1 c mixed nuts (sliced almonds, pecans, walnuts
1 c arugula
2 tbsp avocado oil
1-2 tbsp pure maple syrup
1 tsp coconut sugar
1 tsp ceylon cinnamon
1 tsp pumpkin spice
½ tsp nutmeg
Sea salt

Optional:
Vegan mozzarella cheese crumbles or feta cheese

1. Preheat oven to 400 degrees. Prepare baking sheet with parchment paper.
2. Skin and pit the butternut squash and then cut into 1" squares. Spread evenly over the baking sheet.
3. In a small bowl, mix avocado oil, maple syrup, coconut sugar and spices. Brush the squash on both sides until all pieces are covered with the sweet mixture.
4. Use remainder of the mixture and cover the mixed nuts. Spread nuts on baking sheet as well.
5. Bake for 30-40 minutes (until soft and browning), flipping halfway.
6. Remove baking sheet and allow squash / nuts to cool.
7. Add squash and nuts to a large bowl and mix in arugula and vegan cheese crumbles. Drizzle with a little avocado oil if needed.

<u>Meal ideas:</u>

On the side of a meal as a savory and sweet salad, enjoy alone as a treat, bring as a thanksgiving or christmas side.

Quinoa Tabbouleh

2 c cooked quinoa
1 c sprouted chickpeas
1 cucumber
1 tomato
1/4 c fresh minced parsley or cilantro leaves
Olive oil
Fresh lemon juice
Sea salt
Pepper

Prepare and dice veggies finely. Mix all ingredients together and dress with olive oil and freshly squeezed lemon juice until wettened, according to your taste. Sprinkle sea salt and pepper on top.

Did you know that quinoa is not a grain, but a seed? Quinoa is a great plant-based source of protein as it contains all 9 essential amino acids - making it a complete protein. It is a great gluten-free alternative to those who struggle with gluten or with grains. Quinoa is high in fiber and low

on the glycemic index, making it a great food for those who struggle with blood-sugar.

Baked Sweet Potato

3 ways

Bake your sweet potatoes at 400 degrees for 30-60 minutes (depending on size). Stab holes before baking and place right on the rack for best results. I prefer mine to be quite soft because they are sweeter! So I bake mine longer.

Baked Potato with Chili

Cut baked potato in half and cover with 1 c of vegetarian chili (see recipe), and drizzle with cashew cream.

Cinnamon Baked Potato

Cut sweet potato in half and dress with a little coconut oil, nut butter, cinnamon and sea salt.

Mashed Sweet Potato

Scoop sweet potato out of it's skin and into a bowl. Smash with a fork and mix in nut milk, coconut oil, and dust with nutritional yeast or cinnamon. Serve as a side to a main course or with veggies on top.

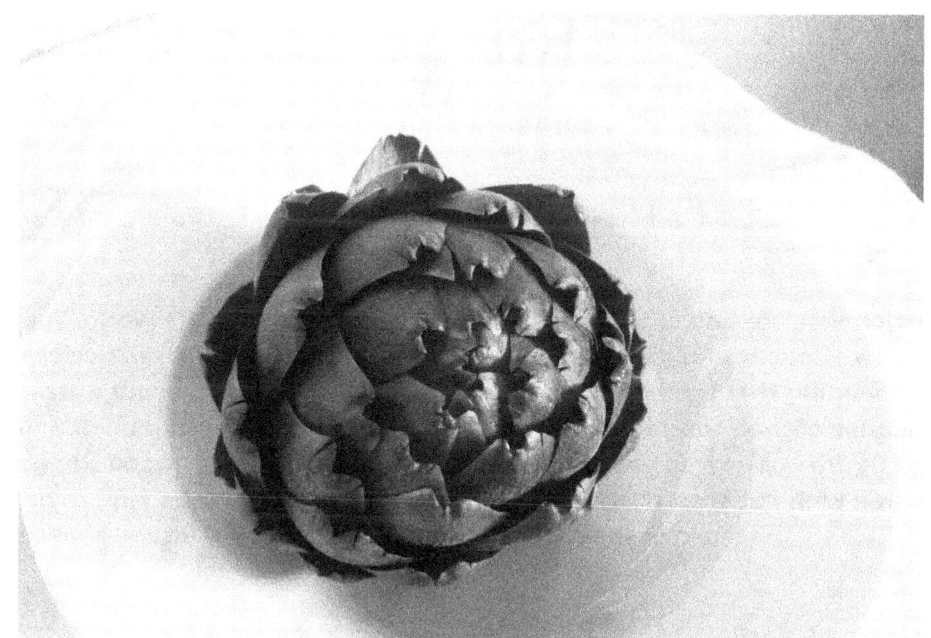

Artichoke Leaves & Heart

1 large organic artichoke

Optional:
Olive oil and fresh crushed garlic mixed and set aside as a dipping sauce

1. Wash your artichoke and cut off the stem about ½ inch from the base.
2. Prepare a large pot with water and bring to a rolling boil, then reduce to a medium-low simmer.
3. Place your artichoke in the pot and cover, allowing to simmer for about 30-45 minutes. You will know it's done with you can stick a fork into the stem and it feels quite soft with no resistance.
4. Remove from heat and allow to cool. Remove from pot and squeeze lightly to discard of any water in the leaves.

How to eat:
Peel off one leaf at a time and examine. You will see the base of the leaf (opposite to the side with a spike) has a "meaty" texture. Place the leaf in your mouth with the inside facing your tongue and use your bottom teeth to scrape the meat from the artichoke leaf from about halfway, down to the base.

Do this until you have reached the "heart" of the artichoke. Once you reach the heart, the fine hairs in the center are not edible. Using a knife, (or your thumb) scrape and discard out all the fine hairs until only the base, heart, and stem remain. This is all edible, and it's the best part! Enjoy!

<u>Meal ideas:</u>
Enjoy alone, dipped in olive oil and garlic. Chop up artichoke heart and stir into a pasta dish.

Artichokes are one of the most antioxidant rich foods in the world. They are also extremely high in dietary fiber and are a natural prebiotic, meaning that the artichoke is food for healthy bacteria in our guts. Because of their tough exterior and interesting form they can be difficult to figure out how to eat, but just like everything in life, all good things come with patience and hard work. This food is highly satisfying to eat because of the care and time it requires to eat it.

Baked or Steamed Veggies

Making a batch of cooked veggies 1-2 a week is an easy way to implement them into your meals when you're short on time. Choose a variety of your favorite vegetables such as:

Carrots
Sweet Potato
Beets
Parsnips
Russet, red, golden potato
Zucchini
Yellow Squash
Broccoli
Cauliflower
Peppers
Squashes

You'll also need
Avocado oil
Spices: Nutritional yeast, sea salt, pepper, cayenne pepper, basil, oregano, rosemary, thyme or parsley are some options.

1. Preheat your oven to 400 degrees. Prepare a baking sheet with parchment paper.
2. Chop your veggies of choice into long strips or round chip-shapes. Place in a bowl and drizzle with a little avocado oil, tossing until completely covered. Add desired spices and toss until covered.
3. Spread flat on the baking sheet and bake in the oven for 25-45 minutes (depending on if a leafy or root veggie) or until softened and lightly browned. Flip halfway.
4. Use right away or save in glass container in the fridge.

To steam, use a steaming basket in a pot of simmering water and allow to sit in steam basket with lid on pot for 25-30 minutes. Steaming will better preserve nutrients, but is more difficult to spice for flavor. I recommend steaming when possible but baking is better than no veggies!

Meal ideas:

Dip into hummus or guacamole, build a hearty buddha bowl, cut up into a salad, put in a wrap, serve over mashed potatoes, as a side to black bean burgers, freeze and throw into smoothies.

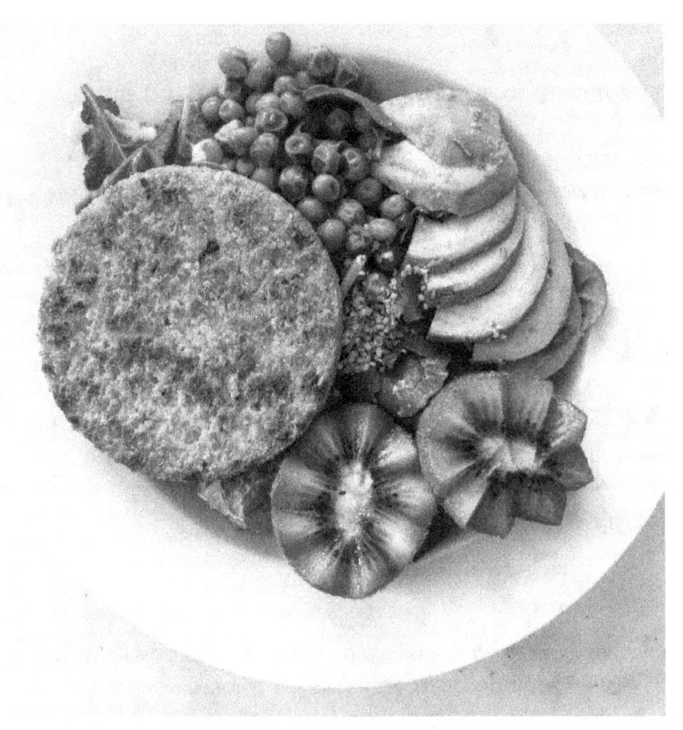

MEALS / SOUPS / SALADS

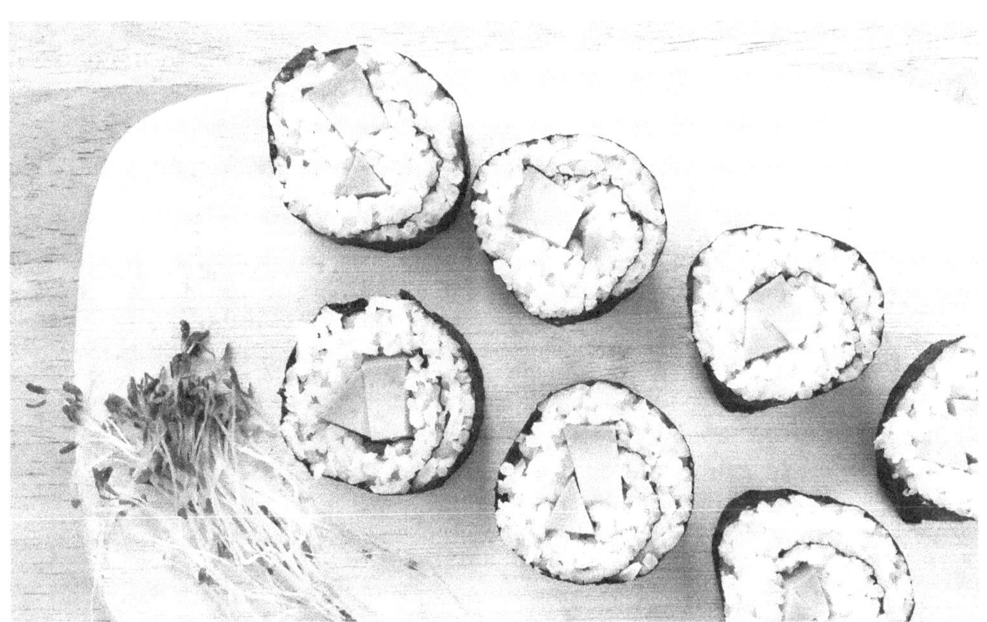

Plant-based Nori Rolls

1 c cooked short grain sushi rice
2 sheets seaweed nori
1 avocado
1 carrot sliced thinly
1 cucumber sliced thinly

1. Take a thin, clean dish towel and soak in water. Wring it out as much as you can until it is only damp, not dripping wet.
2. Lay towel out on the counter, and lay 1 nori sheet on it, rough side up
3. Scoop rice on to nori sheet and spread it out evenly in a thin layer, covering the sheet except for the last inch of the side farthest away from you.
4. Lay your toppings in an even line horizontally close to the edge that is nearest you.
5. Begin slowly lifting the towel and curling the edge nearest you over the toppings. Press down gently, firmly, and evenly from the outside edges to the inside.
6. Use fingers to curl the edge in and slowly roll it forward. Use the towel to help you lift, and press the roll every 1/2 - 1 inch.

7. Once you get to the edge, use a drip of water and slide it along the portion of the nori sheet that doesn't have rice. Finish curling the roll until it has covered the final edge. Press again.
8. The roll should be sturdy enough to cut! Wet your knife and slice in 1 inch rolls, wetting your knife between every cut to avoid ripping the nori sheet.
9. Dip in tamari sauce or wasabi and enjoy!

Seaweed is a very nourishing food for the body. All sea vegetables are an especially helpful food for those with thyroid problems and pregnant/nursing women. They are very high in chlorophyll which is a natural and powerful detoxifier. Sea vegetables are also high in iodine which is not found easily in other foods. Seaweed contains essential fatty acids, is anti-cancerous, and helps to heal the skin.

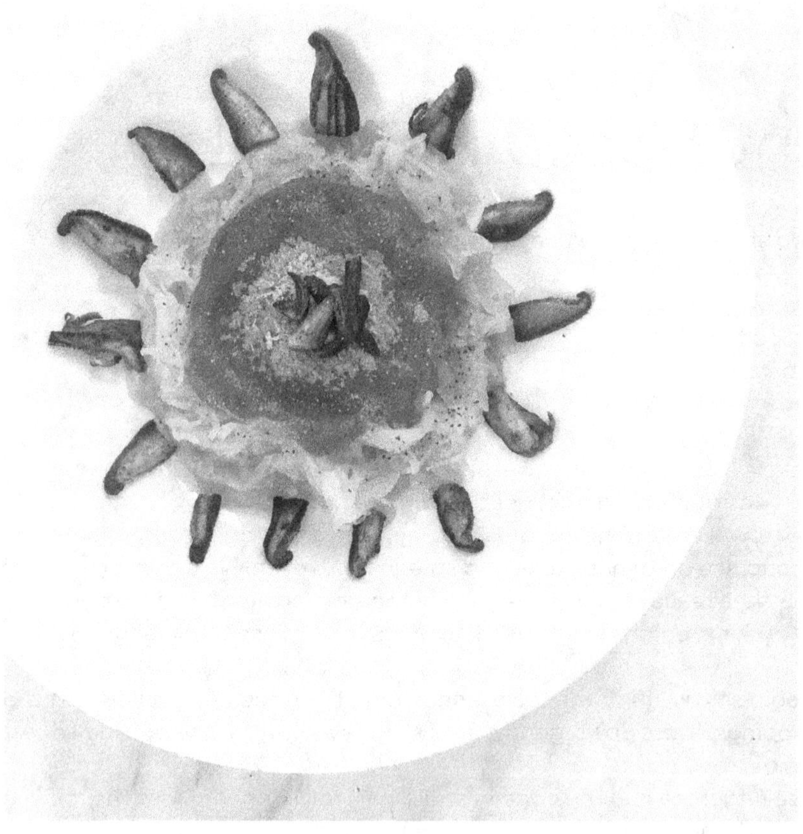

Spaghetti Squash with Lentil Marinara

1 large spaghetti squash
1.5 c plain marinara sauce
1/2 c lentils, cooked
1/4 onion, diced
3 cloves garlic, crushed
1-2 c chopped veggies of choice
        (I like to do red peppers, zucchini, broccoli, or mushrooms)
½ tsp each of spices like basil, oregano, red pepper flakes, and nutritional yeast
Sea salt
Pepper
Avocado oil

1. Preheat oven to 400 degrees
2. Prepare squash by stabbing holes in it with a fork, and microwave it for 1-2 mins, (this softens it enough to cut). Cut in half lengthwise and scoop out seeds with a spoon.
3. Brush oil evenly over squash and salt and pepper it lightly.
4. Using a glass dish, place squash halves face up in the pan, and place in the oven for 45 minutes.
5. Meanwhile, cook lentils by adding 2 c of water and bringing to a boil, then reducing and simmering on low heat for about 15-20 minutes.
6. Add veggies to a saucepan and saute on medium-low heat until aromatic.
7. Add sauce, spice and lentils to the saucepan and simmer for about 5 minutes and reduce to low until squash is ready.
8. Remove squash from the oven and allow to cool. Fork away at the edges to get a "spaghetti" consistency.
9. Pour lentil marinara into the squash boat sprinkle nutritional yeast on top!

This meal is another husband favorite! This is a great upgrade for one of america's favorite comfort foods. Both of my kids have also loved spaghetti squash as babies and as a toddler.

Vegetarian Goulash

2-3 c cooked fusilli/macaroni shaped quinoa or brown rice noodles
1 jar of marinara or spaghetti sauce
1-2 c chopped veggies such as:
Zucchini
Yellow squash
Tomato
Peppers
Mushrooms
Carrots
1 tbsp nutritional yeast
Sea salt
Pepper
½ c cashew parmesan

Optional spices:
Paprika, basil, oregano, turmeric

Add cooked noodles to a pot and stir in sauce, spices and chopped veggies. Simmer on low for 5 minutes or until combined. Serve warm and sprinkle cashew parmesan on top.

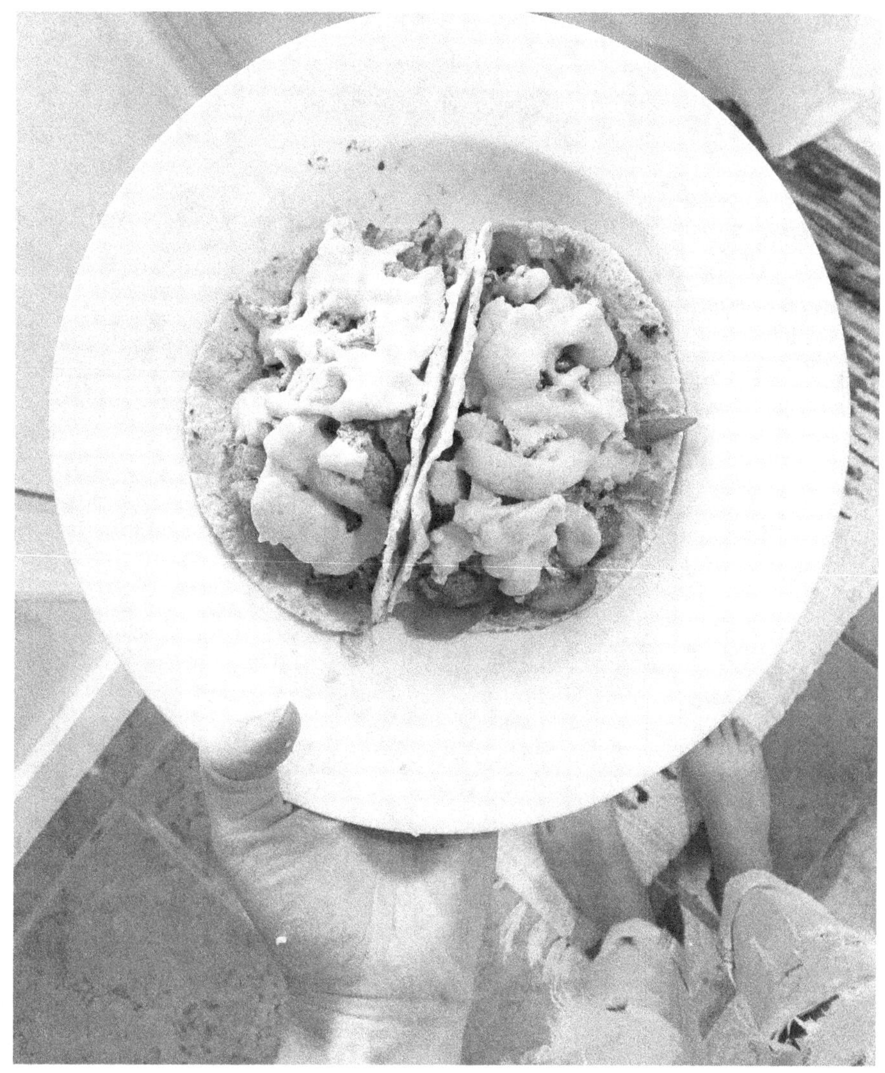

Plant Tacos

1 head of cauliflower

1 c chickpeas

1 c cooked quinoa

1 c fresh veggies (peppers, onions, mushrooms)

1 c black beans

1 ripe avocado, sliced

1 c mac n' cheez sauce
or cashew cream (see recipes)

6-10 sprouted organic corn or whole wheat tortillas
Avocado oil
1 lime

<u>Taco seasoning</u>
About ½-1 tsp of each:
Nutritional yeast
Coconut sugar
Cayenne pepper
Red pepper flakes
Turmeric
Cumin
Sea salt
Pepper

<u>Salsa</u>
1 fresh tomato
½ onion
¼ c fresh cilantro

1. Preheat oven to 400 degrees. Prepare a baking sheet with parchment paper and set aside.
2. Cut head of cauliflower into small florets and place into a bag with chickpeas. Drizzle avocado oil and add taco seasoning and then shake until everything is covered/combined. Pour contents onto the baking sheet and spread evenly. Place in oven to bake for 30 minutes, flipping halfway.

3. Cut fresh veggies into strips/chunks and place in a saucepan. Sprinkle with any remaining taco seasoning. Saute on medium-low heat until aromatic then set aside and cover.

4. Prepare the salsa by chopping or mincing up the ingredients and mixing together with a spoon. Set aside.

5. Prepare the mac n' cheez sauce (which doubles as "Nacho cheez") or cashew cream. Leave as is, or add taco seasoning and a squeeze of lime to the cashew cream to get a creamy chipotle-type sauce.

6. Prepare tacos by placing your tortilla on a place, and piling on quinoa, beans, veggies, your "taco meat" (cauliflower/chickpeas), and adding some slice avocado, salsa and a drizzle of creamy cheez of your choice on top!

Leave out tortillas and make a taco-bowl, make a taco salad by adding ingredients over freshly chopped romaine lettuce and using cream sauce as a dressing, add ingredients into a large tortilla and roll into a burrito

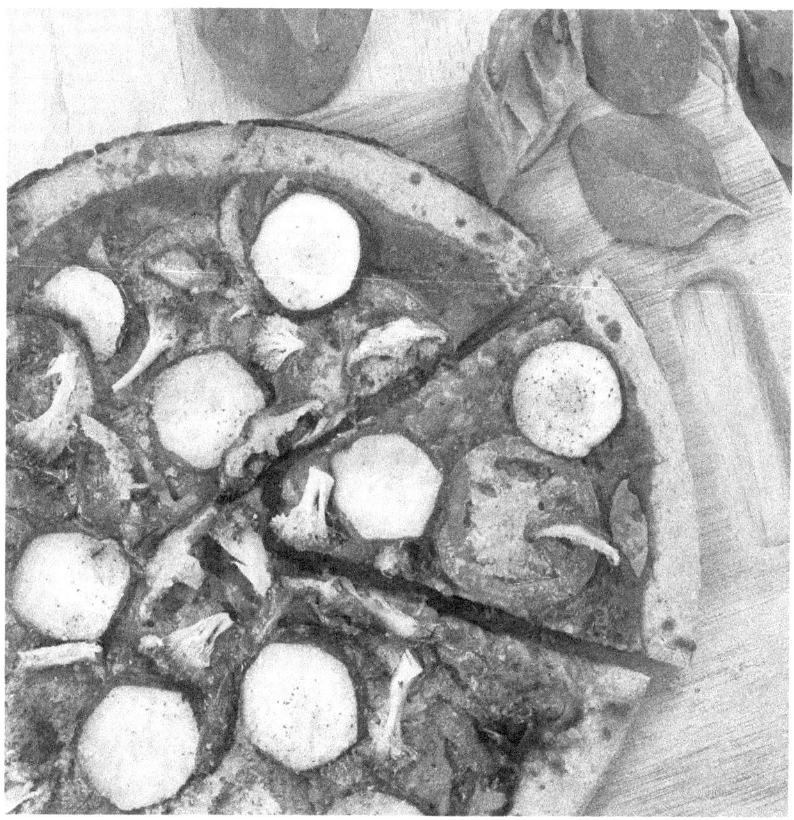

Veg Pizza

2 pizza crusts (cauliflower, gluten free, or whole wheat)*
1 c marinara sauce
1 c mushrooms
1 c zucchini
1 c red/green peppers
½ c red onion

½ c broccoli
½ c spinach
1 c mac n' cheez sauce
    Or cashew cream (see recipes)
½ c cashew parm (see recipe)

*I typically use Bob's Red Mill gluten free pizza crust mix, or Trader Joe's Cauliflower pizza crust in the freezer section. Haven't perfected a crust recipe yet!

1. Preheat oven to 425 degrees. Bake your crusts of choice.
2. Wash and prepare veggies by slicing thinly. Prepare mac n' cheez or cashew cream sauce and cashew parm (see recipes) as well!
3. Prepare pizza by spreading a layer of marinara sauce over your crusts. Place veggies on pizza according to your liking. Drizzle with creamy cheez sauce of choice and sprinkle with cashew parm.
4. Bake for an additional 10-15 minutes (according to recipe for your crust).
5. Allow to cool and then slice with a pizza cutter into triangles.

<u>Meal ideas:</u>

Dip into vegan ranch dressing, if not plant-based enjoy recipe with a sprinkle of mozzarella cheese under your veggies.

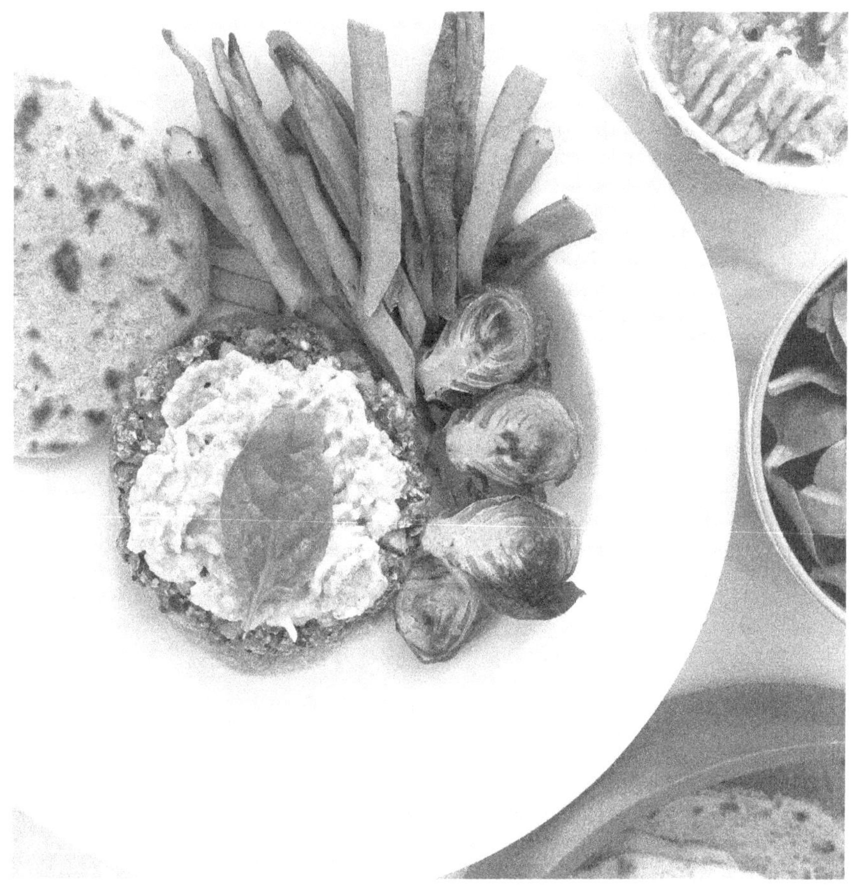

Black Bean Burgers

1.5 c organic black beans (or 1 can)
1 c instant oats
1/2 onion
1 celery stalk
2 tbsp ground flax seed
1/4 c nut milk
¼ tsp each of spices such as:
  sea salt, garlic powder, onion powder, nutritional yeast,
  black pepper and cayenne pepper

1. Preheat oven to 350 degrees and line baking sheet with parchment paper.

2. Add 2 tbsp ground flax seed and 3 tbsp water into a small bowl, mix and allow to sit for a few minutes.
3. In a small bowl combine oats and spices.
4. Pour black beans into another bowl and mash (it's easiest if you use your hands). Add oats and veggies and using hands mix until combined. Slowly add almond milk to get desired consistency. You want it to feel moist but not too sticky. Add more oats to dry, and milk to wetten.
5. Taste and adjust spices to your liking. Use hands to form patties and place on parchment paper.
6. Bake for 20 minutes flipping halfway. Burgers are done when outside is crispy!

<u>Meal ideas:</u>

Serve on a whole wheat bun with avocado, tomato, mushrooms, onions and greens. Serve over a bed of fresh greens and add chopped tomato, avocado, and dress with a vegan ranch dressing. Break up and use as bulk in breakfast burritos, wraps, or tacos.

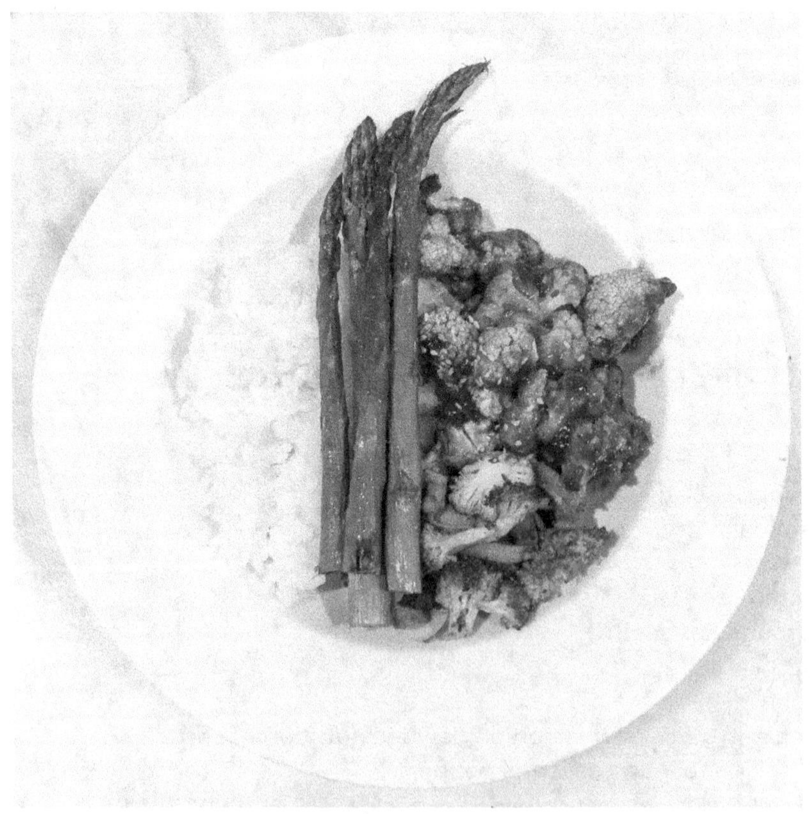

Cauliflower Teriyaki

2 c cooked basmati rice
1 head of cauliflower
1 c veggies such as:
Peppers
Broccoli
Zucchini/yellow squash
Mushrooms
Snow peas
Green beans
½ - 1 c teriyaki sauce or orange chicken sauce
¼ c green onions
2 tbsp organic corn starch or arrowroot flour/starch
1 tbsp sesame seeds
Avocado oil
Garlic powder
Sea salt
Pepper

1. Preheat oven to 400 degrees. Prepare a baking sheet with parchment paper.
2. Cut up cauliflower florets into small bite sized pieces. Put into a bag and drizzle with avocado oil, shaking bag until all florets are covered. Pour corn starch into the bag and shake until all surfaces are covered.
3. Pour florets out onto the baking sheet and sprinkle with sea salt and pepper. Bake for 30-45 minutes flipping halfway. Florets should be crispy and browning. Broil on high for 2-3 minutes at the end to get desired crisp.
4. While cauliflower is baking, slice veggies and saute on medium low heat until aromatic. Set aside and cover with a lid.
5. Remove cauliflower from the oven and allow to cool (on a cooling rack if possible) for about 10 minutes. Add cauliflower into a saucepan and cover in teriyaki sauce. Stir and simmer on low heat until sauce thickens and becomes absorbed by the cornstarch. Cauliflower should closely resemble the look of orange chicken.
6. Serve cauliflower and veggies over a bed of rice and sprinkle green onions and sesame seeds on top.

Meal ideas:

Use any asian sauce and use as healthy alternative to breaded chicken, put cauliflower into lettuce wraps

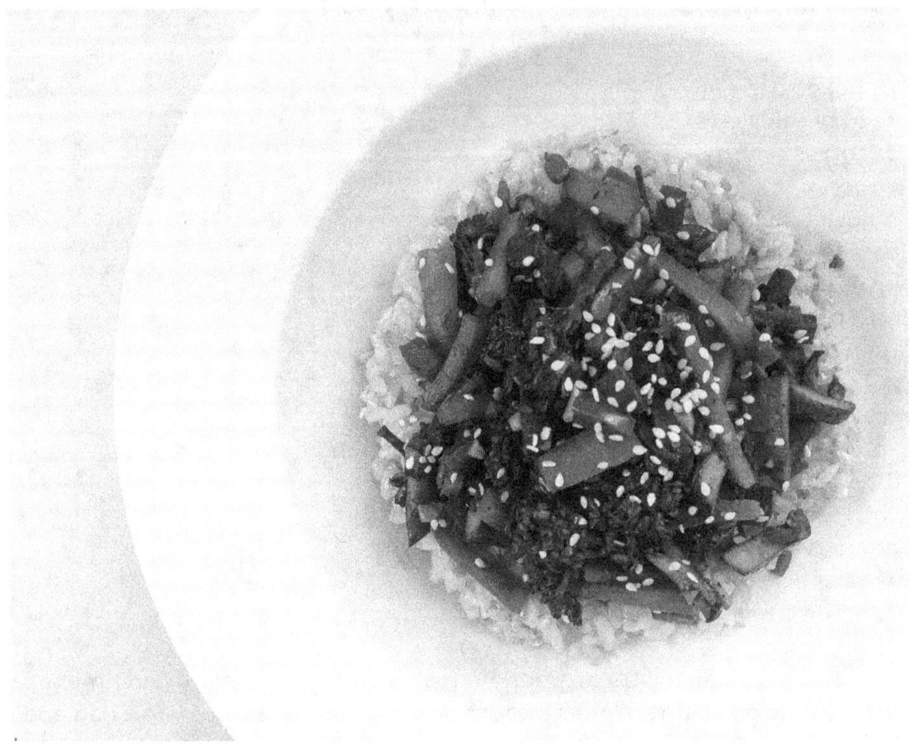

Coconut Cashew Stir Fry

1 c short grain brown rice
2-3 c roughly chopped veggies such as:
Red/green pepper
Broccoli
Zucchini
Mushrooms
Green beans
Onions
Carrots
¼ c chopped cashews
2 tbsp Coconut Aminos (or tamari sauce)
1 tbsp unsweetened coconut shreds (optional)

1. Add rice to a pot with 2 c filtered water. Bring to a boil and then lower to a simmer and cook for 45 minutes.
2. In a saucepan, add all desired veggies and sauteed in coconut aminos on medium-low heat until aromatic. Try not to overcook.
3. Serve veggies over rice and sprinkle chopped cashews and coconut shreds on top!

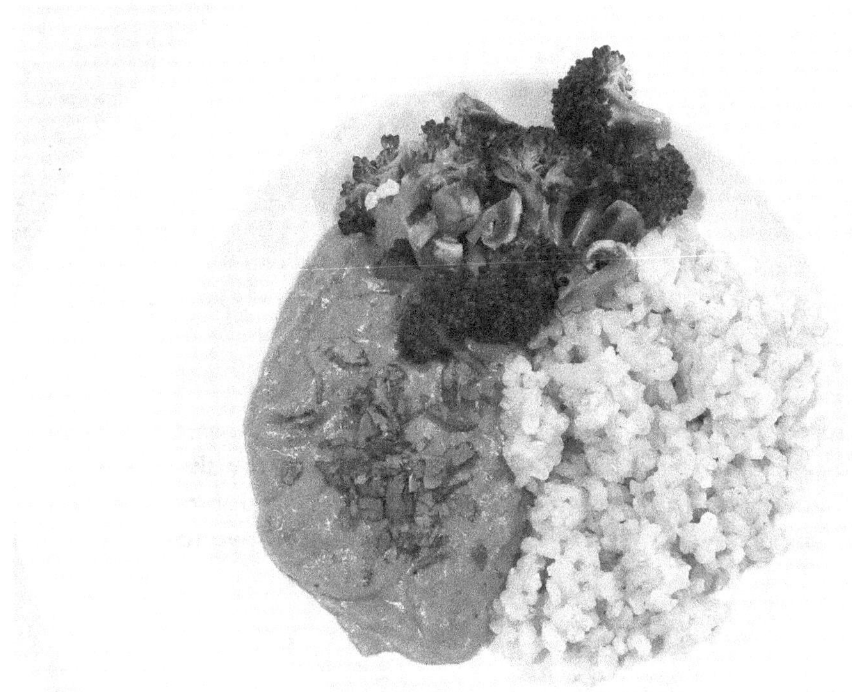

Legume Tikka Masala

2 c cooked basmati rice
1 can organic full fat coconut milk
1.5 c (or 1 can) of tomato sauce (with chunks)
1 c lentils or 1.5 c chickpeas
¼ c cashews, soaked*
2 tsp lemon juice
2 tsp garam masala spice

1 tsp cumin
½ tsp sea salt
¼ tsp turmeric
¼ tsp ginger
⅛ tsp cayenne pepper
1 tsp pure maple syrup
5 cloves of garlic, crushed
1 sprig cilantro

*cashews will give it a thicker consistency, and more "bulk". Consider trying sauce without it first, and adding if you find it to be too runny. Mixture will thicken with simmering especially with addition of cashews.

1. Add all ingredients (except lentils/chickpeas) into a high speed blender. Blend until combined, and add to a pot. You can add dry lentils to the sauce and simmer for 20 minutes (or until lentils are soft) or you can cook separately and combine, as you would with chickpeas, near the end. Allow sauce to simmer either way for about 20 minutes on low heat.
2. Serve over basmati rice and garnish with minced cilantro.

Cilantro is a great herb for detoxing from heavy metals and killing off pathogens. If you struggle with a chronic health condition, one of these issues may be at the root cause! Consider the addition of cilantro to your diet every day to help the body to naturally remove toxins and heal.

Burrito Bowls

2 c cooked short grain brown rice
2 c chopped veggies such as
Red/green peppers
Red onions
Zucchini
Mushrooms
1 c sprouted, cooked black beans (or canned)
2 ripe avocados
½ c cashew cream (see recipe)
Sea salt
Black pepper

Cayenne pepper

1. Prepare veggies by roughly chopping. You can lightly saute on medium-low heat until aromatic or keep raw.
2. Build burrito bowls by adding all ingredients into 2 seperate bowls and adding sliced avocado on top, as well as drizzling cashew cream. Add spices according to taste.

<u>Meal ideas:</u>

Serve in whole wheat tortillas for a true burrito. Serve over a bed of greens and add some cayenne and lime to the cashew cream, using it as a dressing for a burrito salad. Enjoy alone over rice.

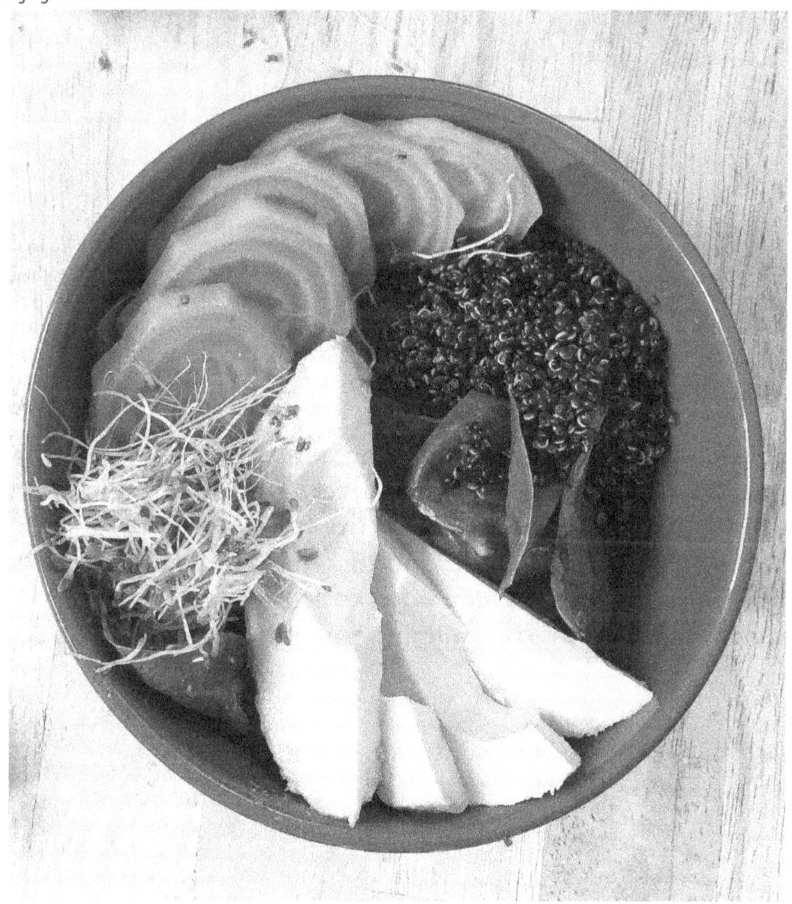

Buddha Bowls

2 c cooked quinoa
1 c sprouted chickpeas (or canned)
½ c steamed red beets
½ c steamed broccoli
½ c lightly steamed spinach
½ c alfalfa sprouts
½ c sunflower seeds or cashews
1 c cashew cream (see recipe)

Place all ingredients in a bowl and drizzle with cashew cream. Makes 2 buddha bowls!

<u>Meal ideas:</u>

This recipe is just a template. Play around and exchange quinoa for other grains like rice, exchange chickpeas for other legumes like lentils/beans, and use any veggies you'd like from your fridge.

The "buddha" bowl is meant to bring about feelings of peace and tranquility. As a powerful spiritual teacher, buddha embodied the attributes of peace and compassion. The more plants we eat, the more compassionate we are to animals and the more we become connected to the earth. I love using a buddha bowl as a very plant-dense meal and I always feel the spiritual enlightenment it offers me to do so.

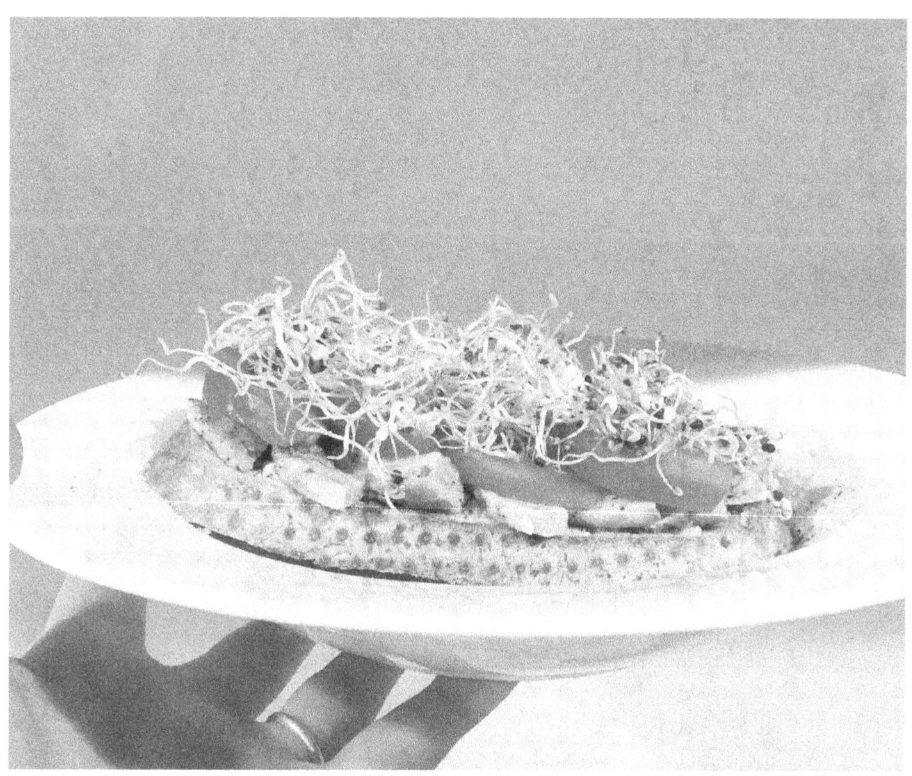

Balsamic Avocado Toast

2 slices of whole wheat or gluten free sourdough toast
1 avocado
1 heirloom tomato
½ c alfalfa sprouts
2 tsp balsamic vinegar
1 tsp olive oil
Pink himalayan sea salt
Black pepper
Nutritional yeast

Toast sourdough to desired crispiness. Slice avocado and tomato and set aside.
Top toast with avocado, spices, olive oil, tomato, and sprouts then drizzle balsamic
vinegar over the top.

Miso Soup

4 c filtered water
1 c organic non-gmo firm tofu
1 c broccoli florets
½ c baby bok choy
½ c mushrooms
¼ c green onions
2 tbsp miso paste
2 cloves garlic, crushed
1 tsp ginger
½ tsp sea salt
¼ tsp turmeric
Black pepper

Optional:
1 package of rice or millet ramen-style noodles (cooked), 1 sheet of seaweed nori

1. Bring water to a low boil in a pot and reduce to a simmer. Slice veggies and tofu into small chunks according to your liking. Add tofu, veggies, and spices (but not miso!) to the water and allow to simmer on low heat for about 15-20 minutes or until veggies begin to soften.
2. In a small bowl, stir miso in a little bit of water (so it is runny and less of a paste).
3. Remove pot from heat and stir in miso mixture.
4. Stir in ramen-style noodles and seaweed nori strips if desired or serve as is! Sprinkle green onions over top.

Meal ideas:

With ramen noodles, as a sipping broth, to accompany plant-based sushi or a stir-fry.

Miso is a nourishing food for the body for many reasons. First, because it is a fermented food it is high in enzymes and beneficial bacteria to help heal and strengthen the gut. This also means it is beneficial for boosting the immune system, and improving digestion. Miso is also a source of complete protein, and is high in minerals and vitamins.

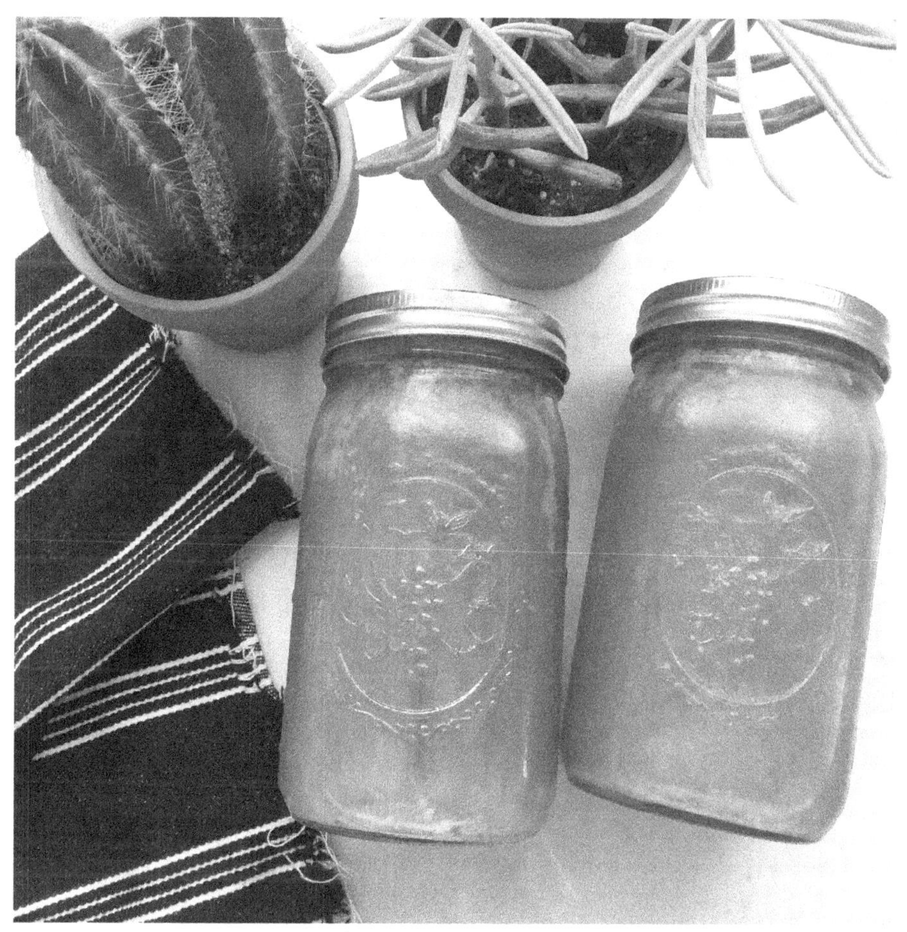

Healing Bone Broth

Bones of 2 whole organic chickens
7-8 c of filtered/purified water
1.5 tbsp organic apple cider vinegar with "the mother"
1 yellow or white onion (cut into 4 chunks with skin still on)
5 cloves of garlic, chopped
1 tsp sea salt
1 tsp garlic powder
1/4 tsp black pepper

Optional:

You can also add scraps of any of your favorite vegetables, such as carrots, potatoes, veggie skins/ends, etc... It will raise the nutrient profile and sulfur level - but it can also affect the taste. I prefer to keep it simple and add stuff in later.

1. It is best if your bones come from chickens that were roasted in the oven at 400 degrees F for that savory taste. If you made them in a crock pot or get them raw, simply bake the bones at 400 for 30-45 minutes or until golden brown.
2. Place all ingredients into a crock pot. Use enough water to just cover the bones and onions, etc.
3. Simmer on low heat for 24-48 hours. (I usually do 24, I find it is sufficient for chicken bones. Beef bones will require 48 hours.)
4. Let cool, strain out remnants and collect broth into a bowl. Pour into glass mason jars. You may have small chunks of skin/fat/garlic which is fine and normal.
5. It will remain good in the fridge for 7-10 days, and last up to 6 months in the freezer.

To drink, NEVER warm the broth up in the microwave. Doing so can denature the proteins and essential nutrients. Always warm up in a pot before drinking. If your broth has fat and gelatin at the top, you can scrape it off - however it will often dissolve once warmed so you don't need to worry.

<u>Meal ideas:</u>

Use as a base for any homemade soup requiring a broth, sip alone for a gut healing tonic, use in place of oil to saute veggies

Bone broth has been around since ancient times. Our ancestors were known to use the scraps of the animals they would hunt for food and simmer their bones, feet, fat, tendons, marrow and cartilage for a healing broth. Today, we can replicate this ancestral practice and bring ourselves the same healing benefits. By low simmering the bones, we draw out the collagen/gelatin, regenerative proteins such as l-glutamine, glycine and proline and minerals present in this part of the animal. Collagen is not made by the body and cannot be found in plant foods. Bone broth is extremely healing to the gut lining. I found that drinking bone broth on a regular basis was one of the most helpful and healing foods in reversing my autoimmune disease and digestive problems. It is a remedy tried and true for thousands of years. The concept of eating "chicken noodle soup"

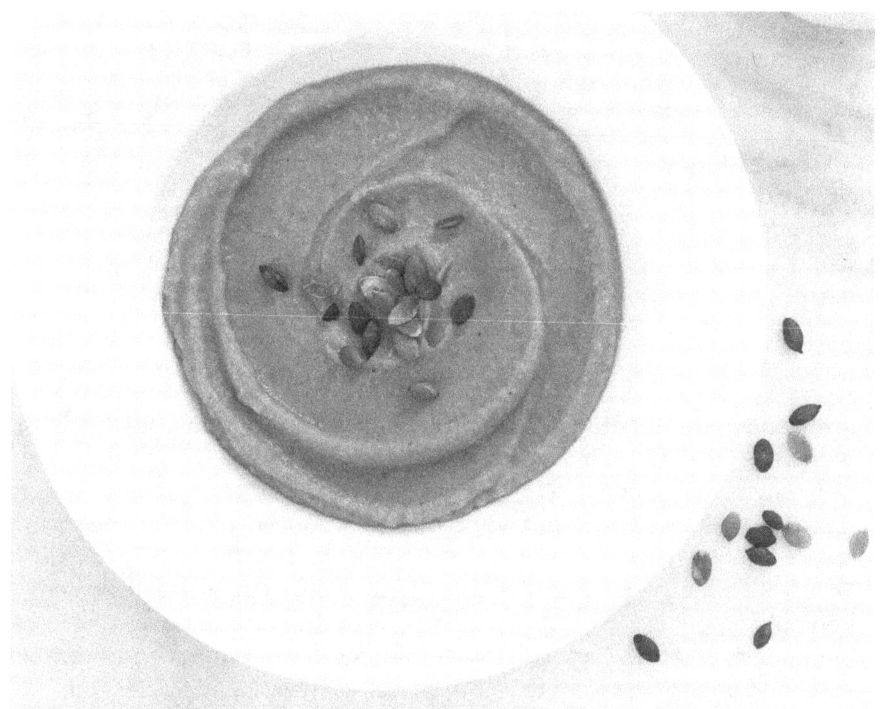

Butternut Sweet Potato soup

1 butternut squash
2 small sweet potatoes (or 1 large)
1 large carrot
1 c nut milk
1 c filtered water
2 tbsp maple syrup
1 tbsp nutritional yeast
1 tbsp ceylon cinnamon
1 tsp pumpkin spice
½ tsp ginger
½ tsp nutmeg

½ tsp turmeric
¼ tsp clove
Sea salt
Black pepper
Avocado oil

Topping:
Pumpkin seeds
Sunflower seeds
Sliced almonds
Avocado oil
Cinnamon
Sea salt

1. Preheat oven to 400 degrees. Cut butternut squash lengthwise and scoop out seeds. Lay face up in a glass dish. Also add sweet potatoes and carrot to the dish. Brush with avocado oil.
2. Bake for 45-60 minutes (depending on size of squash) or until all veggies are soft.
3. Scoop out squash with a spoon, as well as sweet potatoes (leaving skins behind) and put in a high speed blender with the carrot. Add all other ingredients and blend on high for 1-3 minutes or until smooth and combined.
4. Taste and add more spices to liking, as well as more liquid for desired consistency.
5. Pour into a saucepan and warm on low heat.
6. Put nuts and seeds for topping in an oven safe dish or baking sheet and lightly brush with oil and sprinkle with salt and cinnamon. Broil on high heat for 1-2 minutes or until lightly browned.
7. Serve soup with toppings sprinkled over top.

Butternut squash is a timeless and cozy fall food with great health benefits. It is high in potassium, with 1 cup offering more than a banana. It also contains vitamin e, vitamin c, vitamin a and b vitamins, as well as magnesium and manganese. This is also a great first food for introducing a baby to solids.

Split Pea Soup

1 16 oz package (1 lb) dried green split peas, rinsed
3 celery ribs
2 large carrots
2 small potatoes
1 onion
2 cloves garlic
6 c organic vegetable broth
1 tsp sea salt
1 tsp black pepper
1 tsp parsley
1 bay leaf
Sesame seeds

1. Rinse split peas and veggies, and dice all veggies to desired size. Put all ingredients in a slow cooker or pot and stir to combine.
2. Cover and cook on low for 7-8 hours or high for 3-4 hours if in a crock pot. Bring to a boil then reduce to a simmer for about 1.5-2 hours.
3. Halfway through cooking time, remove and discard bay leaf.
4. Serve warm, and garnish with sesame seeds for a nutty undertone.

Creamy Vegetarian Chili

2 cans of diced tomatoes
1 can of roasted diced tomatoes
1 can full fat coconut milk
1 can of chili beans
1 can of black beans
1 can of dark red kidney beans
1 can of pinto beans
1 onion
1 red pepper
1 yellow pepper
1 anaheim pepper
1 jalapeno pepper

2 cloves garlic, crushed
1 tbsp cumin
1 tbsp garlic powder
1 tsp red pepper flakes
1 tsp cayenne pepper
1 tsp sea salt
½ tsp black pepper
Avocado oil

Optional:
Use a packet of taco seasoning instead of suggested spices. Leave out coconut milk for a more traditional chili recipe.

1. Wash and prepare produce, then mince into small chunks. For the hotter peppers mince and small as you can. Add all veggies & garlic into a pot and saute until softened and aromatic.
2. Add all canned ingredients into a crockpot and add veggies and spices as well. Mix until combined. Taste and adjust spices as necessary for desired taste. Add water if you want a more soup-like consistency.
3. Cook in the crock pot on low for 6 hours or high for 2-3 hours. If you don't have a crockpot, simmer on medium-low in a large pot for about 1 hour.
4. Serve warm with sliced avocado and cashew cream on top.

<u>Meal ideas:</u>

Serve over a baked sweet potato, add to mac n' cheez (see recipe) for chili mac, crumble some pulp crackers over it for more texture

Cayenne pepper is a strong herb, with even stronger medicinal benefits! Cayenne is nourishing to almost every system of the body. It is a powerful healing herb for the heart, powerful enough that a good dose of cayenne can stop a heart attack. The regular consumption of cayenne will help to heal the gut lining. Anywhere that applied, cayenne will bring antibodies to the area. It is also a powerful herb for purifying the blood stream and supporting the bodies natural detox processes.

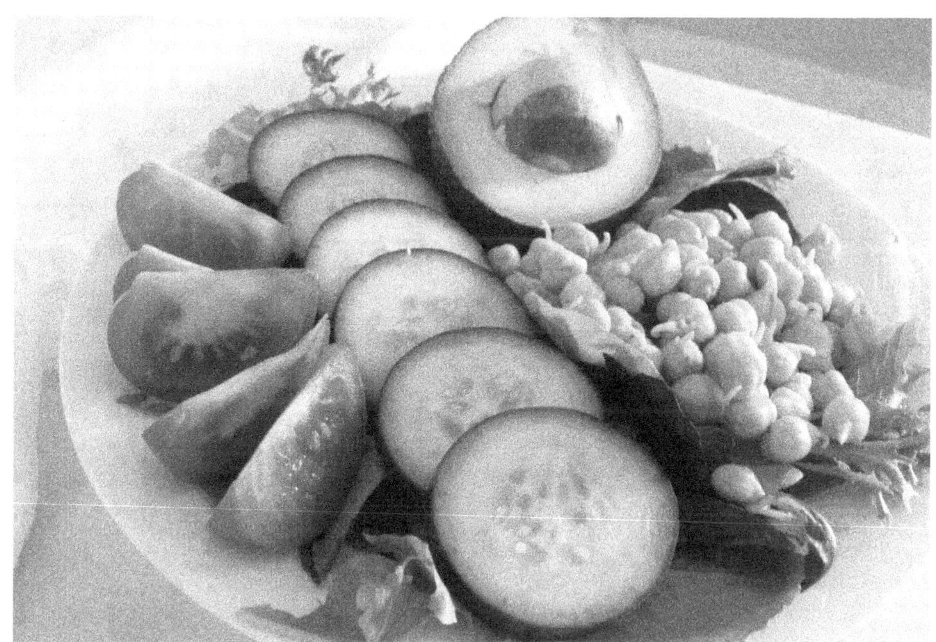

Chickpea Salad

2 c mixed greens (spinach, kale, chard, arugula)
½ c sprouted chickpeas (or canned)
½ avocado
¼ c english cucumber
¼ c tomato
¼ c grated carrot
¼ c alfalfa sprouts
1 tbsp sunflower seeds
1 tbsp olive oil
1 tbsp fresh lemon juice
Sea salt
Pepper

1. Rinse and prepare fresh produce. Slice veggies to desired size.
2. Drizzle greens with olive oil and massage leaves with your hands until fully covered with oil.
3. Add all other ingredients to bed of greens and drizzle with lemon juice and spice according to taste.

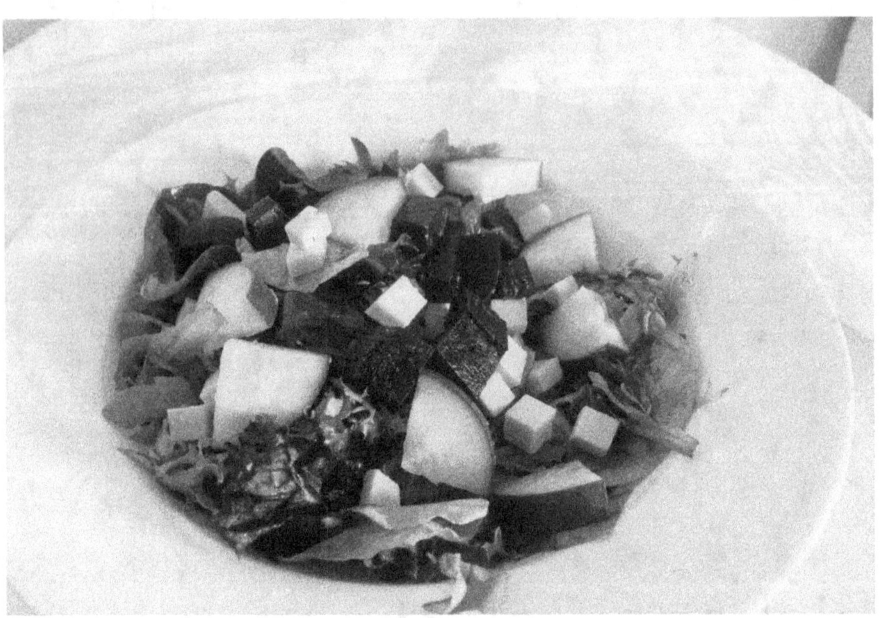

Beet & Cheez Salad

2 c mixed greens
½ c beets, steamed (golden or red)
¼ c cucumbers or zucchini
¼ c microgreens or sprouts
2 tbsp vegan mozzarella cheez (I like myokos brand) or feta
2 tbsp sliced almonds
1 tbsp olive oil
1 tbsp balsamic vinegar
Sea salt
Pepper

1. Rinse and prepare fresh produce. Slice veggies to desired size.
2. Drizzle greens with olive oil and massage leaves with hands until fully covered with oil.
3. Add all other ingredients to bed of greens and drizzle with balsamic vinegar and spice according to taste.

Raw Garden Salad

2 c mixed greens
      (arugula and dandelion greens are great to add)
¼ c carrots
¼ c radishes
¼ c celery or cucumber
¼ c cherry/grape tomatoes
2 tbsp microgreens
Creamy Tahini dressing (see recipe)

1. Rise and prepare fresh produce. Slice veggies to desired size.
2. Drizzle greens with dressing and use spoons to toss until combined.
3. Add other ingredients to bed of greens and enjoy!

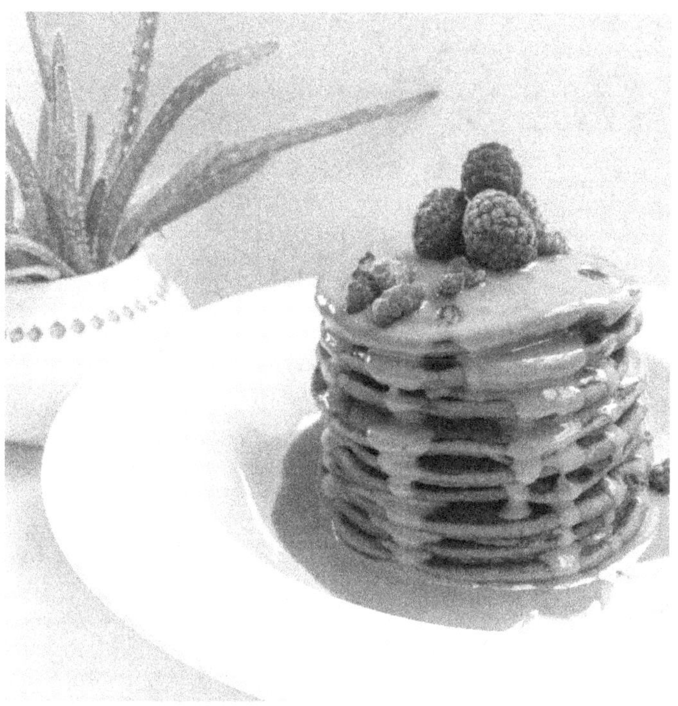

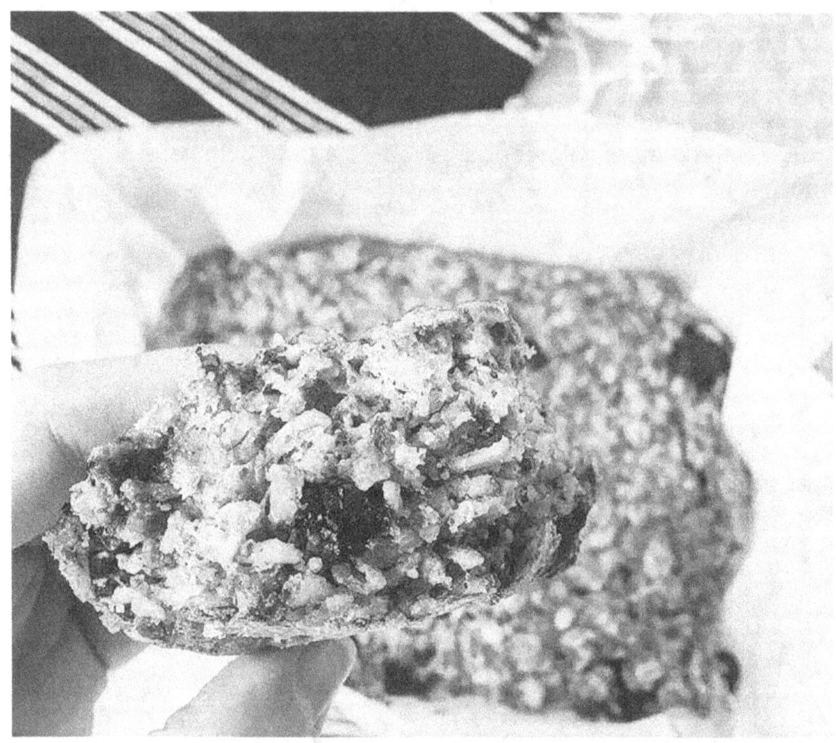

Blueberry Oat Bake

2 c traditional rolled oats
2 overripe bananas
1 flax egg (or egg)
1 c nut milk
1/2 c nut butter
2 tbsp coconut oil, melted
2 tbsp ground flax seed
1/2 tsp baking powder
1/2 tsp baking soda

1/2 tsp vanilla extract
1/4 tsp sea salt
1 c berries or nuts

1. Preheat oven to 350 degrees. Prepare a square 8x8 or similar sized baking dish by lining it with parchment paper.
2. Mix dry ingredients in a bowl. In a separate bowl mash banana and mix in wet ingredients. Combine wet and dry ingredients and mix until combined.
3. Saute fruit in a saucepan until wilted and stir into the mixture.
4. Pour into baking dish and bake for 45-60 minutes or until toothpick comes out clean.

<u>Meal ideas:</u>

Serve warm for breakfast with nut butter spread on top. Break up and sprinkle over a smoothie bowl. Cut up and freeze for future easy on-the-go breakfast bars.

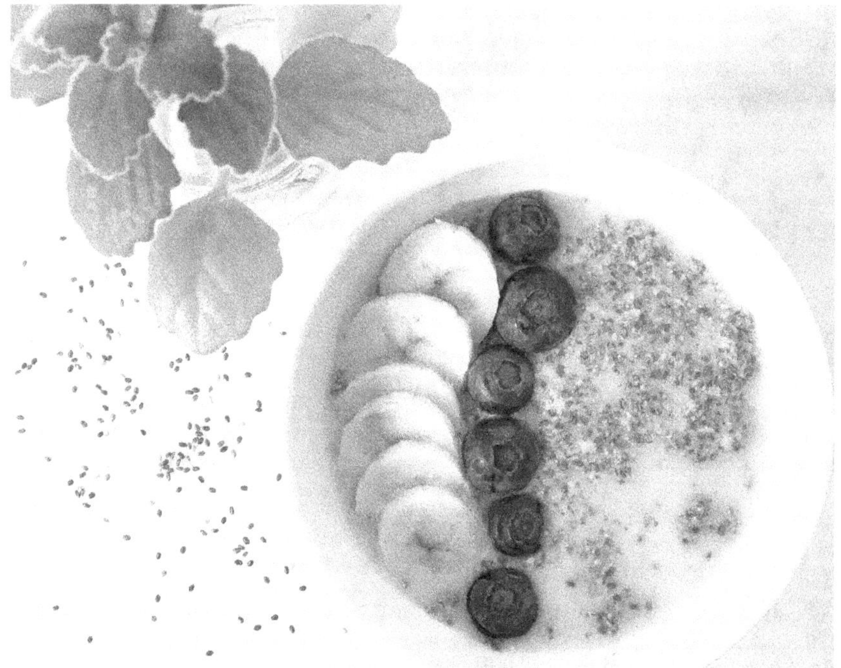

Chia Seed Pudding

3 tbsp organic chia seeds

1-1.5 c nut milk
1 tbsp maple syrup
2 tsp ceylon cinnamon
1 tsp vanilla extract

Add all ingredients together in a mason jar and stir or shake until combined. Set in the fridge overnight for for at least 3 hours.

Meal ideas:

Serve with fruit or granola on top, mixed into a smoothie bowl, blended into a smoothie, add turmeric and more sweetener for an anti-inflammatory boost.

Chia seeds might be small, but they pack a big punch! Chia seeds are high in omega-3 fatty acids, fiber, antioxidants, iron, and calcium. They are a healthy source of protein and fat and help you to feel satiated.

Fruity Overnight Oats

1 c traditional rolled oats
1 tbsp chia seeds
1 tbsp maple syrup
1 tsp ceylon cinnamon
1 tsp vanilla extract
1.5 c nut milk
½ c fruit of choice

1. Add all ingredients in a glass mason jar and stir. Cover with lid and shake until combined.
2. Put in the fridge and allow to sit at least 1 hour or overnight.
3. Enjoy cold with fresh fruit over the top

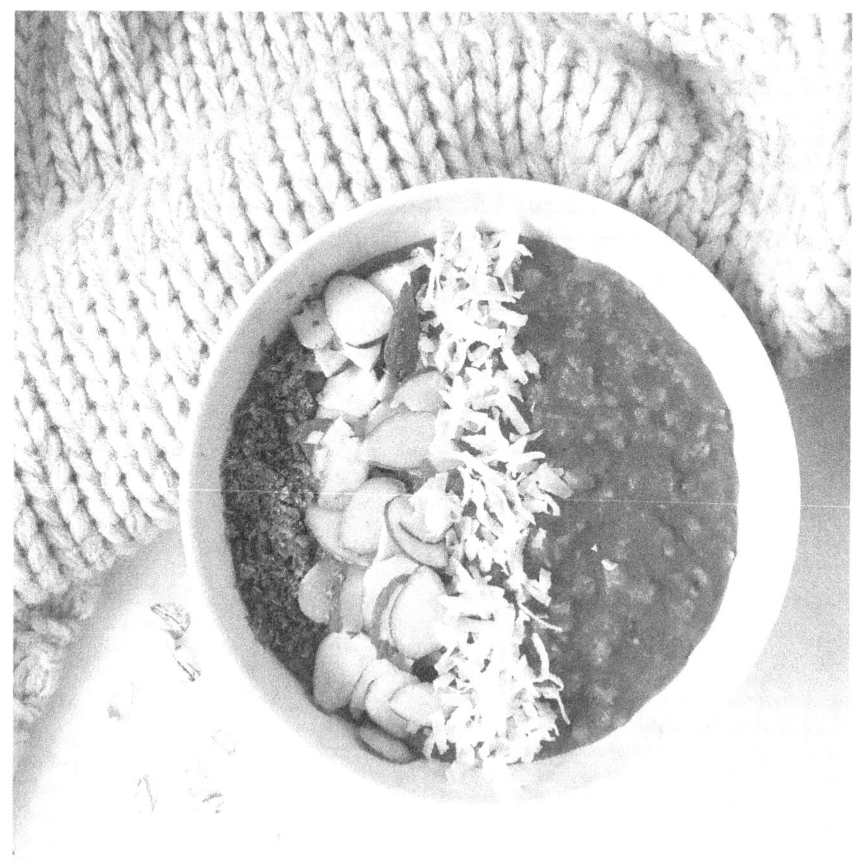

Soultry Overnight Oats

1 c traditional rolled oats
2 tbsp cacao powder
1 tbsp peanut butter
1 tbsp ground flax seed
1 tbsp maple syrup
1 tsp vanilla extract
1.5 c nut milk
½ c cacao nibs, fruit or nuts of choice

1. Add all ingredients in a glass mason jar and stir. Cover with lid and shake until combined.

2. Put in the fridge and allow to sit at least 1 hour or overnight.
3. Enjoy cold with fresh fruit, nuts or cacao nibs on top.

Overnight oats was one of my first "healthy food" recipes I adapted into my life. I find that it's easy to make, tasty, and a good replacement for those who have depended on cereal for breakfast. I also enjoy eating oats as a post-workout to regenerate my muscles. Oats are a great food for boosting milk supply in breastfeeding mothers.

Omelette Cups

6-8 organic pasture-raised eggs
1 c spinach
½ c red/green peppers
½ c zucchini
½ c mushrooms
2 tbsp nutritional yeast
1 tsp garlic powder
½ tsp sea salt
Avocado oil
Pepper
Nut milk

1. Preheat oven to 350 degrees. Grease a muffin tin with avocado oil.
2. Whisk eggs in a large bowl and set aside.
3. Chop veggies to desired size and whisk into eggs along with spices. Add nut milk as desired to increase fluffiness.
4. Pour mixture into muffin tins and bake for about 15-20 minutes or until set in the center.

Meal ideas:

On-the-go easy breakfast, in a breakfast sandwich, broken up into a breakfast burrito with potatoes and cashew cream sauce (see recipe)

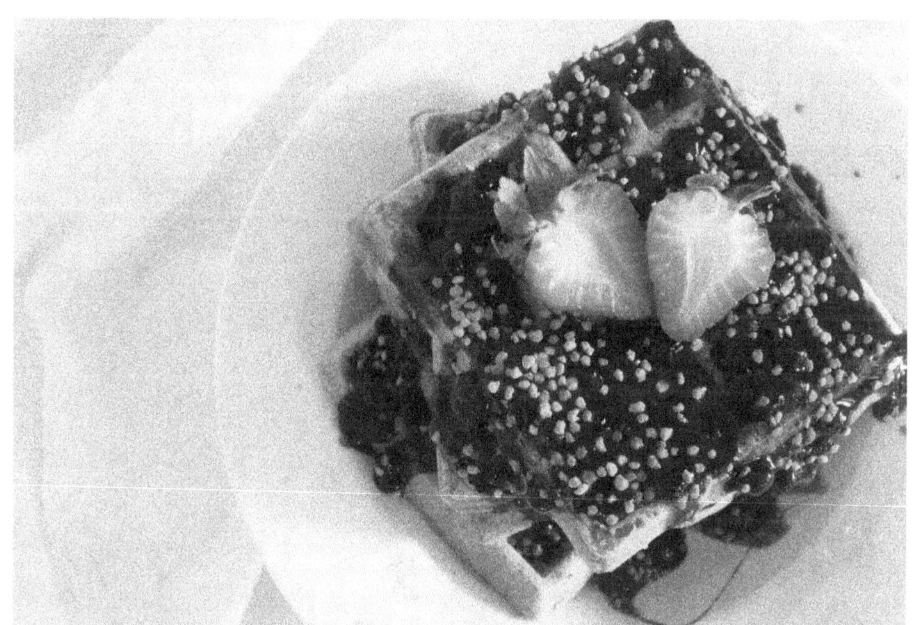

Buckwheat Waffles

1 c gluten free baking flour
½ c buckwheat flour
½ c rolled oats or oat flour
2 flax eggs or organic eggs
1 c nut milk
½ c coconut sugar
2 tbsp coconut oil, melted
½ tsp baking powder
½ tsp baking soda
Pinch sea salt

Plug in waffle iron and allow to heat. Mix dry ingredients in a large bowl. In another bowl, mix wet ingredients. Combine wet and dry and mix until combined. Pour ½-1 c of the mixture onto an oiled waffle iron and cook until crispy!

This recipe is really flexible. You can swap flours in and out as long as you have about 2 cups of flour! I've done oat flour, buckwheat, almond flour, coconut flour, etc. Not all flours are created equal so make sure you don't use more than ½ c almond or coconut and keep oats or a gluten free flour as the main bulking flour. Have fun!

Serving ideas:

Spread raspberry chia jam on top, serve with omelette cups, freeze and put in toaster for a quick on-the-go meal

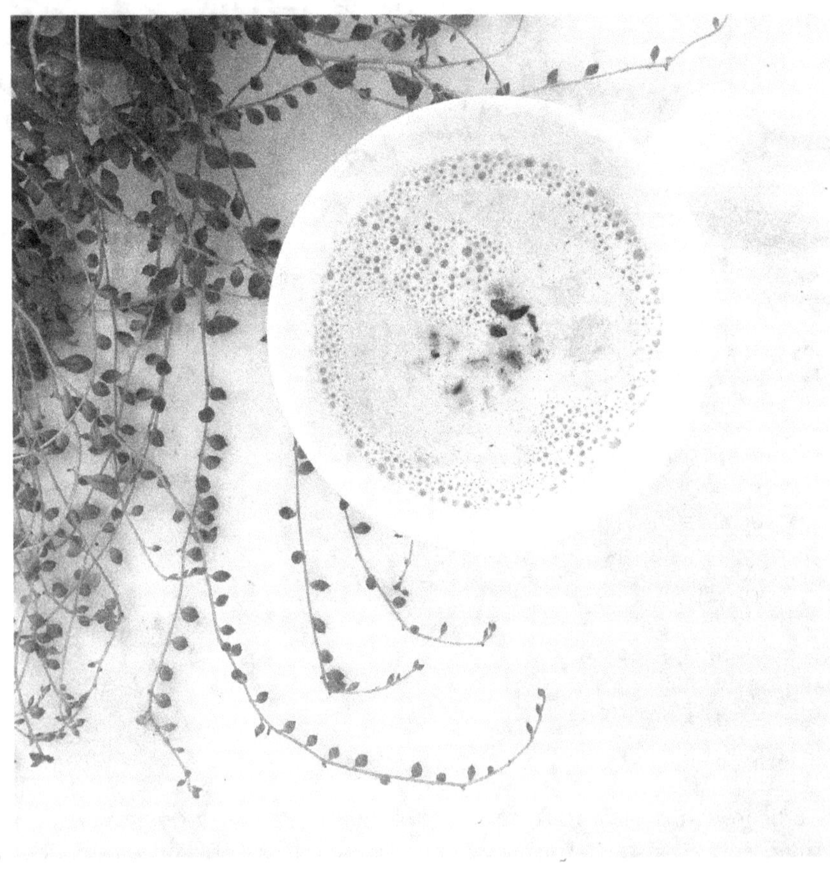

ELIXIRS / TEAS

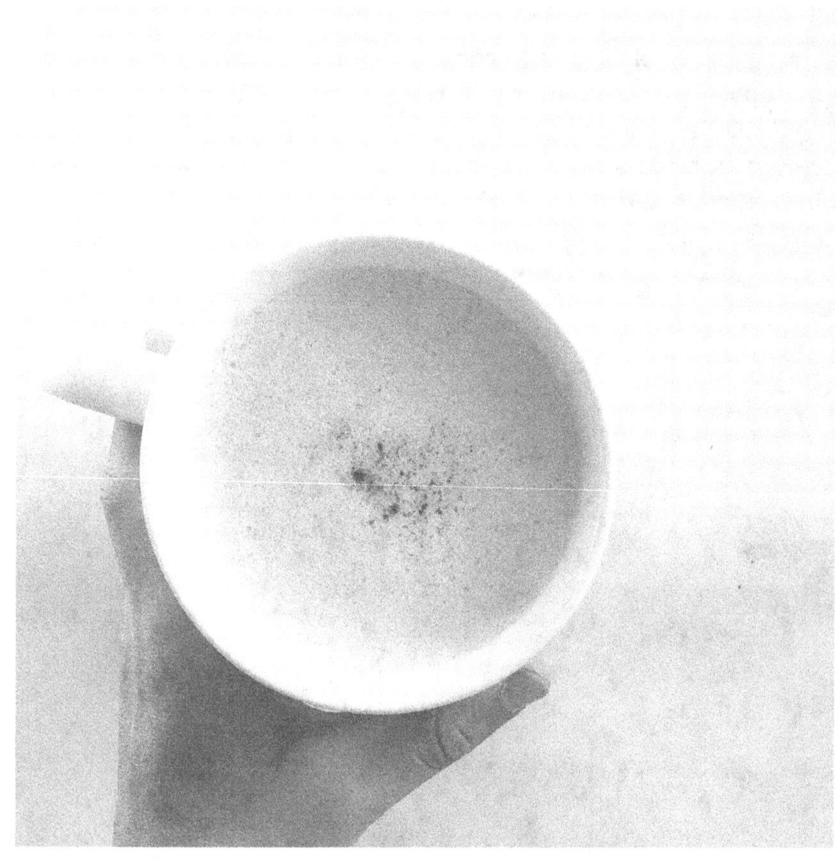

Golden Turmeric Milk

1.5 c plant milk
2 tsp raw honey or maple syrup
¼ - ½ tsp organic turmeric powder
Few dashes organic ceylon cinnamon
Pinch black pepper
Dash vanilla extract

1. Warm plant milk over the stove on medium-low heat. Add ingredients except honey and whisk until combined.
2. Take pan off the stove and whisk in honey at the end before serving.

Turmeric, regarded as a sacred root in India, is a highly anti-inflammatory herb. Studies have shown that it is equally as effective as tylenol and other NSAIDS at reducing pain and inflammation in the body! It is also anti-cancerous, boosts brain function and improves digestion. It is a great aid in healing the gut and reducing anxious feelings. Those who are taking pain killers or struggling with chronic pain may benefit from medicinal doses of Turmeric.

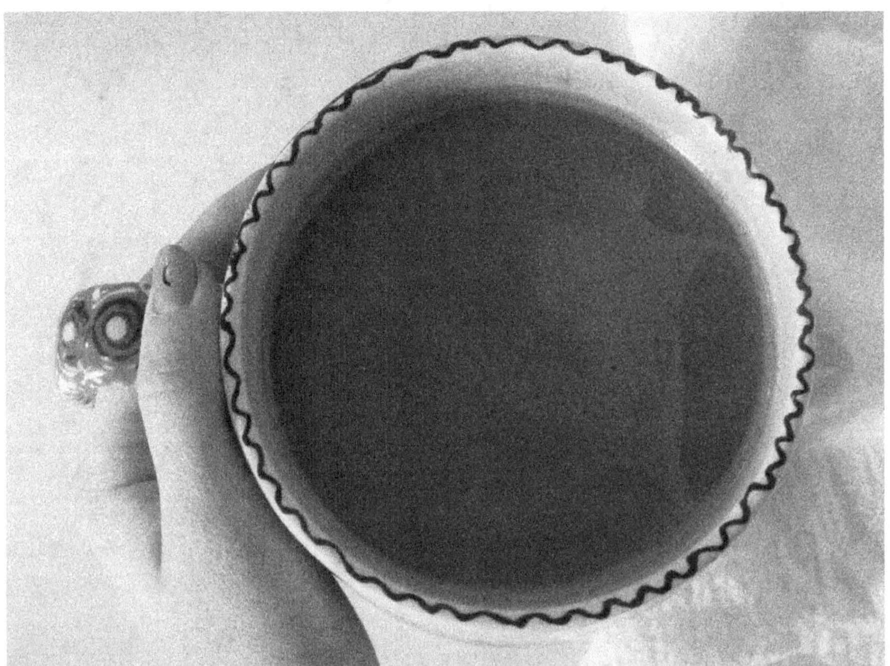

Mushroom Hot Cocoa

1.5 c plant milk
1 tbsp raw cacao powder
1 tbsp raw honey or maple syrup
1 tsp vanilla extract
½ tsp chaga or reishi mushroom powder
Dash sea salt

1. Warm plant milk over the stove on medium-low heat. Add ingredients except honey and whisk until combined.
2. Take pan off the stove and whisk in honey at the end before serving.

Reishi mushroom is the Queen of the Mushrooms. A supreme healer, this herb contains several medicinal constituents. Reishi is best known for its ability to reduce anxiety and improve sleep. It also supports good digestion and purifies the blood. Reishi is adaptogenic in nature, meaning that when it's consumed it adapts to the needs of your body. It also contains trace amounts of psilocybin which is found in high quantities in psychedelic mushrooms, and is currently being studied as a possible treatment for those suffering with mental illnesses. I have used Reishi mushroom for years and can attest to its healing properties.

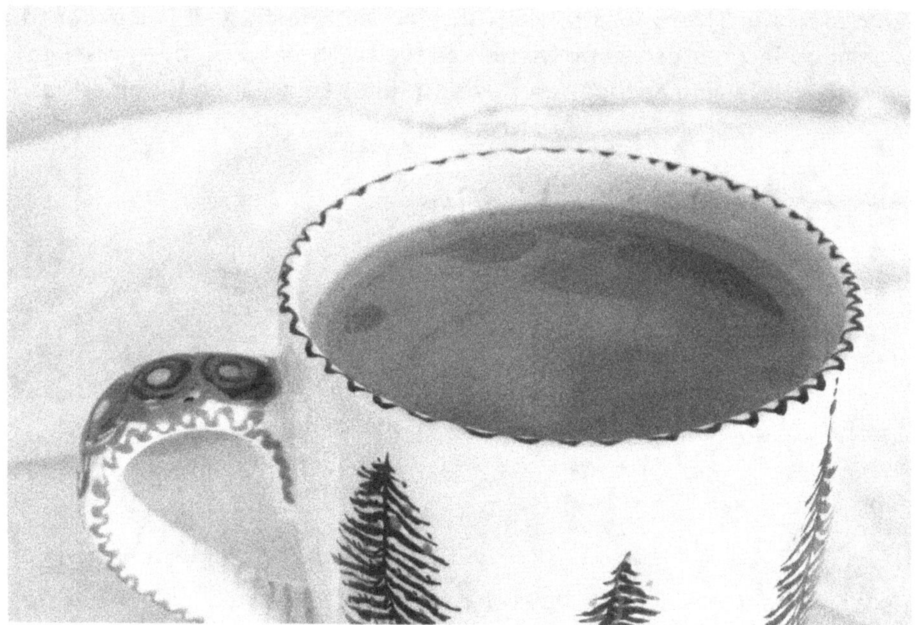

Night Cap Elixir

1.5 c plant milk
1 tbsp raw cacao powder*
1 tbsp raw honey or maple syrup

½ tsp ashwagandha
½ tsp reishi mushroom powder
½ tsp he shou wu powder
Dash ceylon cinnamon

*cacao can be a stimulant for some due to the naturally occurring caffeine , or relaxing to some because of the magnesium and other constituents. If it seems to stimulate you, don't include in your nightcap if drinking before bed.

1. Warm plant milk over the stove on medium-low heat. Add ingredients except honey and whisk until combined.
2. Take pan off the stove and whisk in honey at the end before serving.

Ashwagandha, another adaptogenic herb that anyone can benefit from. This root is especially effective at reducing stress, anxiety, and depression as well as lowering cortisol levels (the stress hormone). Ashwagandha is a powerful healing herb for those struggling with fertility. It is a great tonic for boosting testosterone in men as well as balancing hormones in women. It is also anti-cancerous and helps to balance blood sugar problems.

Moonlight Tonic

1.5 c plant milk
2 tsp raw honey or maple syrup
1 tsp reishi mushroom powder
¼ tsp turmeric
¼ tsp ceylon cinnamon
⅛ tsp ginger
Dash of vanilla extract

1. Warm plant milk over the stove on medium-low heat. Add ingredients except honey and whisk until combined.
2. Take pan off the stove and whisk in honey at the end before serving.

Apple Orange Cider

1 c freshly juiced apple
½ c orange juice
1 tsp apple cider vinegar
½ tsp ceylon cinnamon
Dash nutmeg
Dash clove

Pour apple and orange juice into a pot and simmer on medium-low heat. Add ingredients and whisk together until combined. Serve warm in a mug.

Ceylon cinnamon is a powerful herb, but it is not the regular cinnamon you see on the shelf at the grocery store. Mass produced cinnamon is actually "cassia" cinnamon, which does not have the medicinal benefits of ceylon and it also contains toxins from the processing. Upgrade your cinnamon to ceylon as soon as possible. Ceylon cinnamon has medicinal qualities such as: anti-clotting factors, anti-bacterial/anti-fungal, and it is a powerful blood-sugar regulator. Add this cinnamon to your snacking and it can reduce the blood sugar spike. Ceylon is also anti-inflammatory and helps to boost the immune system.

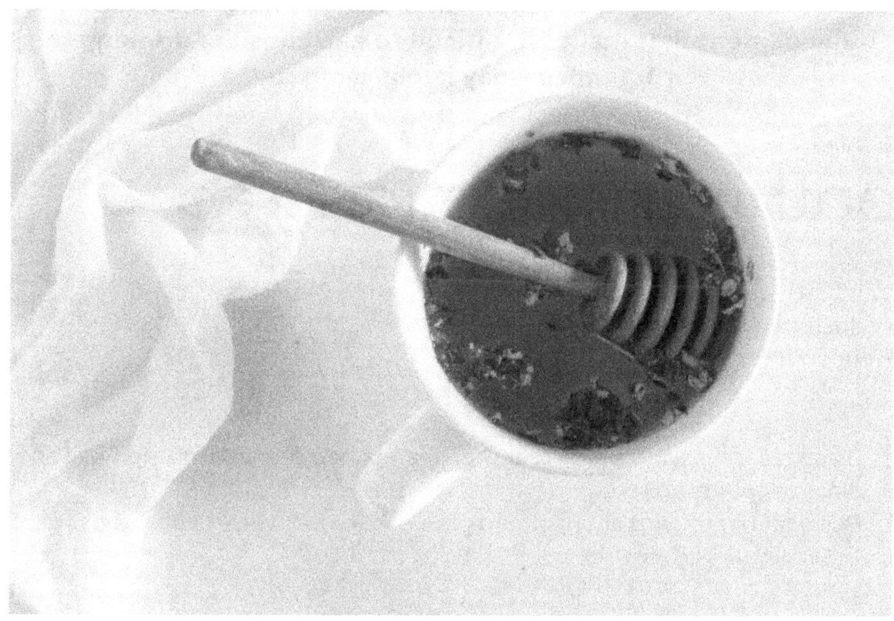

Red Raspberry Leaf Tea

1.5 c purified water
1 tsp wildcrafted red raspberry leaves
1 tsp raw honey (optional)

1. Place tea leaves in a cotton tea bag or stainless steel mesh tea infuser ball and place in your mug.
2. Boil water, remove from heat and pour over tea. Cover and allow to steep for 10-15 minutes or until tepid.
3. Remove tea bag or ball. Stir in raw honey before serving.

Red Raspberry Leaf is nature's prenatal vitamin. For any woman who is trying to get pregnant or is pregnant - you want this herb in your life on a daily basis. Red raspberry leaf also helps to tone the uterus, which can lead to a smoother birth. This herb is extremely high in vitamins and minerals which also makes it great for post-partum mama's and breastfeeding. For everyone else - it is a great multivitamin and electrolyte. If you are struggling with food poisoning, the flu, a cold, or any other ailment that makes it difficult to eat, consider drinking this tea 3-5 times a day in place of food.

Soothing Digestion Tea

1.5 c purified water
1 tsp wildcrafted catnip leaves
1 tsp fennel seeds

1. Place tea leaves and seeds together in a tea bag or mesh infusion ball and place in your mug.
2. Boil water, remove from heat and pour over tea. Cover and allow to steep for 10-15 minutes or until tepid.

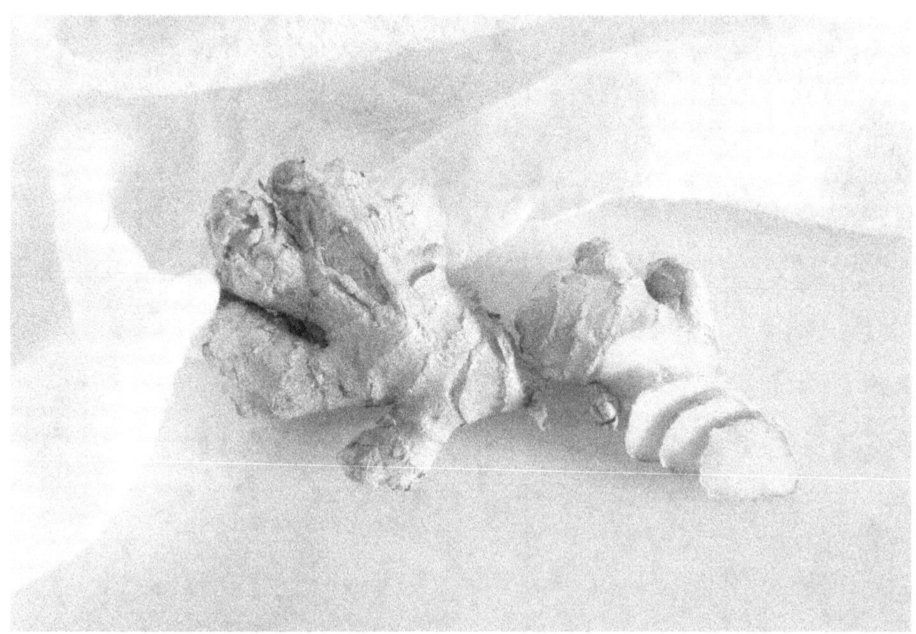

Upset Tummy Tea

1.5 c purified water
1 inch fresh ginger root
1 tsp raw honey

1. Skin the knob of ginger and cut it into slices.
2. Bring water to a boil and then reduce to a simmer, add ginger slices quickly. Simmer on low heat for 20 minutes.
3. Strain out ginger and pour tea into your mug. Stir in raw honey right before serving.
4. You can use the same ginger slices for 1-2 more cups of tea.

Ginger root is one of the best digestive healing herbs available. It is soothing to an upset stomach, reduces bloating and gas, and reduces nausea. It also is highly anti-inflammatory and helps to boost the immune system. This is a great herb to implement into each day for optimal health.

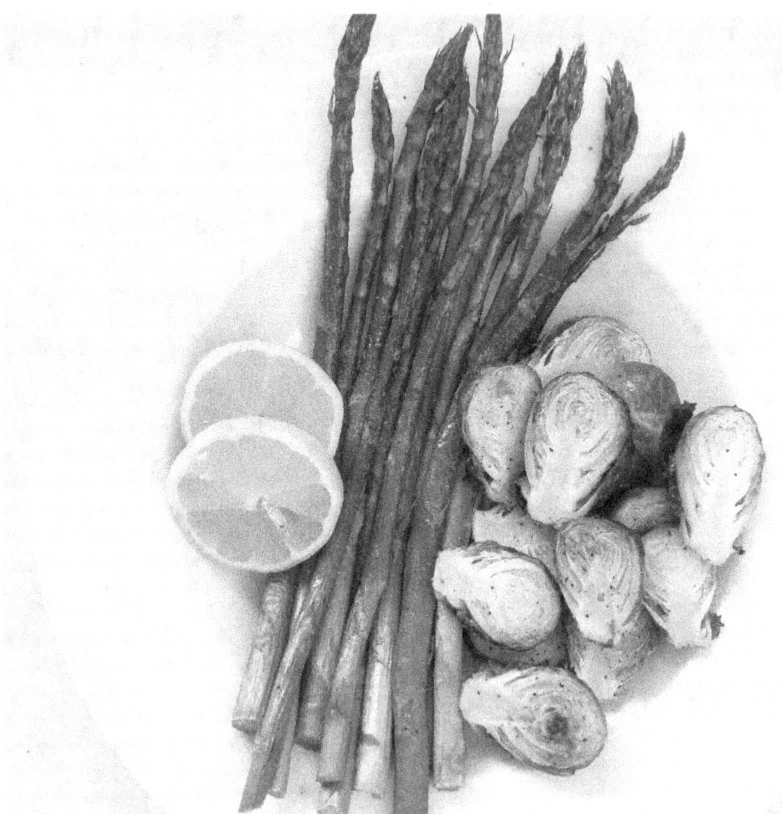

Shopping List

One of the most difficult parts of eating well is knowing what to buy. Most of the recipes I've created use the same basic ingredients! I wanted to create a list of my "staples" that allow me to make most of the recipes in this book, and more! Although some recipes will call for more specific ingredients (like dill pickles need fresh dill which I don't always have laying around), I won't be including every ingredient but just the ones that you'll want to make regular staples. Although the size of your family, your available grocery stores, and your preferences may dictate a different shopping list, feel free to use this as a "starting place" or resource to know what healthfully stocked pantry and fridge can look like.

MY STAPLES

Fruits	Vegetables	Grains/Legumes	Nuts/Seeds	Herbs/Spices	Other
Apple sauce	Artichoke	Black beans (dry or canned)	Alfalfa seeds (to sprout)	Basil	Apple Cider Vinegar
Apples Avocados	Beets		Almond Flour	Black Pepper	Arrowroot Flour
Bananas	Broccoli	Buckwheat flour	Almond butter	Cacao Powder	
Blueberries	Butternut Squash	Chickpeas (dry or canned)	Almonds, raw	Cacao nibs	Avocado Oil
Dates Frozen Cherries	Carrots		Cashews, raw	Cayenne	Balsamic vinegar
	Cauliflower	Flour (whole wheat or gluten-free)	Chia Seeds	Ceylon-Cinnamon	Canned Coconut Milk
Frozen mixed berries	Cucumbers	Lentils	Flax Seeds (whole or ground)	Cilantro	Coconut Aminos
	Golden Potatoes	Quinoa		Clove	
Frozen tropical fruit mix	Kale	Quinoa or brown rice noodles	Hazelnuts	Cumin	Coconut Oil
Grapefruit Lemon	Marinara sauce		Hemp Seeds	Garlic Powder	Coconut Sugar
	Mixed Greens	Rice, basmati	Peanut butter	Garlic, fresh	Coconut flour
Oranges or Orange Juice	Mushrooms	Rice, brown short grain	Pumpkin seeds	Ginger root, fresh	Eggs
	Onion			Ginger spice	Miso paste
Pears	Red Peppers	Rolled Oats	Sunflower seeds	Mustard	Olive Oil
Raspberries	Seaweed		Tahini	Nutmeg	Pure Maple Syrup
Strawberries	Spaghetti Squash		Walnuts	Nutritional yeast	Raw Honey
Any and all fruit!				Parsley	Tamarai Sauce
	Spinach			Red Raspberry Leaves	Unsweetened Shredded Coconut
	Sweet potatoes			Reishi Mushroom	Vegan or real Mozzarella
				Sea Salt	White Wine Vinegar
	Tomato			Turmeric	
	Zucchini			Vanilla Extract	

TOOLS YOU'LL NEED

In order to make many of my recipes you'll want some basic kitchen tools. I'll list all the ones I suggest getting eventually, but I'll list them in order of importance (meaning only the first few are absolutely necessary):

- High speed blender

- Non-toxic cookware

- High quality knives, whisk, spatula

- Mason jars and lids

- Nut milk bag

- Sprouting lid or jar/tray

- Steam basket

- Juicer

- Food processor

- Hand Spiralizer

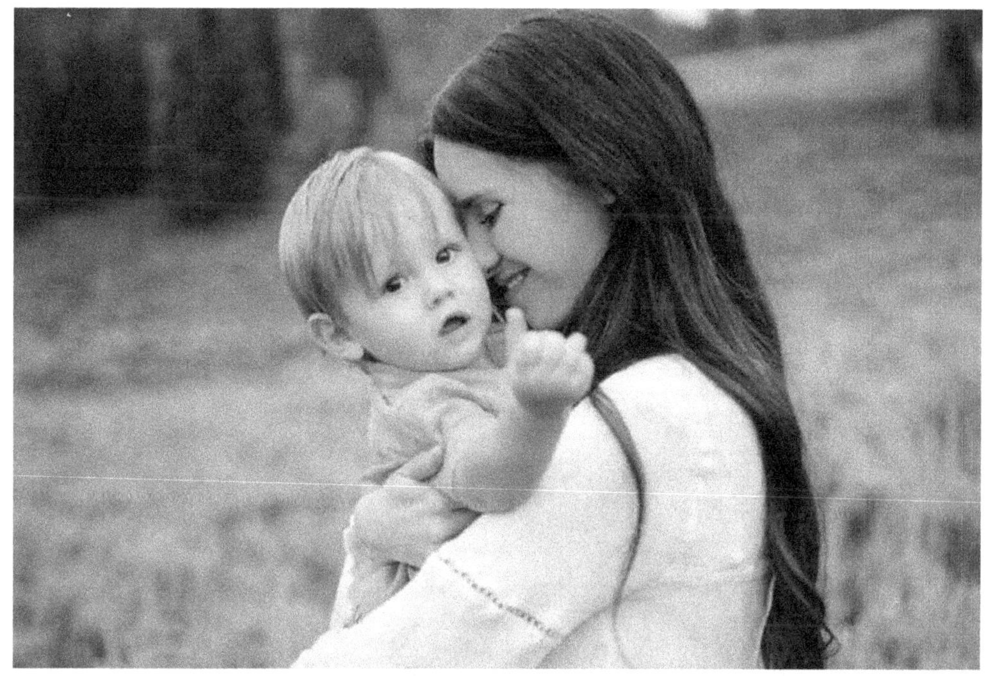

Conclusion

Thank you for sharing this piece of my journey with me! I hope that something you read inspires you to take steps toward loving yourself, improving your health, and knowing where to start. Any time I finish reading a book, whether it's about health or self-help or whatever, I always find myself battling with a decision. My decision is whether I will take what I learned from it and put it to action... Or if I will stay the same, letting the knowledge I gained fade away. It is my greatest wish that anyone who reads this will realize that they can heal their life. It's up to you!

In my personal application of the information I shared with you, I have found a great deal of relief. Our physical body seems complex but it is simple to care for when we nourish it naturally as it was intended. There is so much that goes into our well-being other than the physical. If you're not already, I recommend pairing your interest in improving your physical health with healing mentally and spiritually too. Just as food is powerful in its ability to nourish or damage our bodies, so are our thoughts and beliefs about ourselves. In the last year of my life I have seen that a lot of my disease was founded in my emotional traumas, holding onto negative emotions, and negative self-talk/criticism. Once I started to love myself, love my body, and take a mindful approach to fueling my body is when I have been able to see the greatest improvements. Although this book is primarily focused on nourishing your physical body, I feel I would be amiss if I didn't share the whole picture around what is actually necessary for genuine health. Start loving yourself and loving your body by caring about what you are putting into it. Put it to the test, and I promise you will enjoy all the benefits of the medicinal power of food.

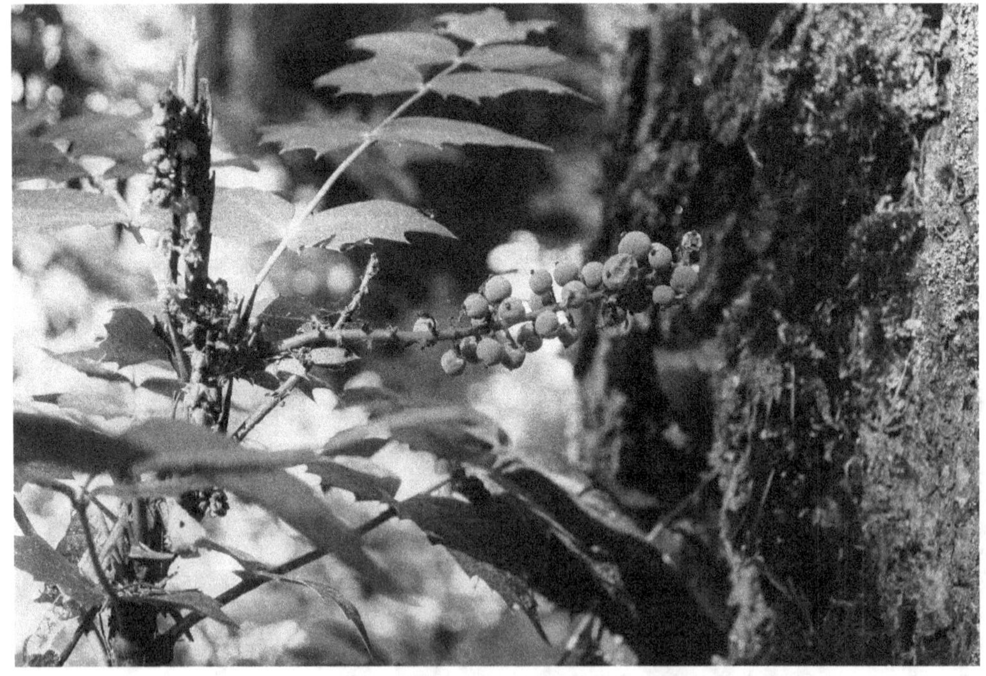

References

1. "Herbal Home Health Care". Dr. John R Christopher.
2. "Just What is the Word of Wisdom?". Dr. John R Christopher.
3. "Prescription for Nutritional Healing" . Phyllis A Bach.
4. "Life Changing Foods". Anthony William.
5. "How to Raise a Healthy Child in Spite of your Doctor". Robert S Mendelsohn
6. "Vitalist vs Atomist". Video lecture by David Christopher, Master Herbalist
7. "You Can Heal your Life". Louise Hay.
8. "Food Irradiation: What you need to know". Food and Drug Administration. https://www.fda.gov/food/resourcesforyou/consumers/ucm261680.htm
9. "What are Sprouts Good For?". Dr. Joseph Mercola. https://foodfacts.mercola.com/sprouts.html
10. "6 Dangers of Conventional Cookware + 4 Best Types Non-Toxic Cookware". Annie Price. https://draxe.com/best-nontoxic-cookware/
11. "Natural Fermentation". Cultures for Health. https://www.culturesforhealth.com/learn/category/natural-fermentation/
12. "Sprouting". Cultures for Health. https://www.culturesforhealth.com/learn/category/sprouting/
13. Butterfly, portrait and family photos by Izabelle Caldwell.
14. Melissa Chappells book of FAVES. Melissa Chappell. www.freshmelissa.com
15. "The best cruelty free mac and 'cheese'". Laura Davis. http://laurasveganeats.blogspot.com/2015/11/the-best-cruelty-free-mac-cheese.html